12-15 Lead ECG Interpretation

New to the fourth edition of this workbook are the Quick Response or QR codes. These codes, as seen below, link to websites or videos. If you have a Smartphone or tablet computer with a camera you can download a free QR scanner. When you hold the scanner over top of the code it will take you to a link related to the content on that page of the book such as a webpage with additional text or video.

Paramedic Tutor Blog:
http://paramedictutor.wordpress.com
Videos links are under the eLearner tab

Paramedic Tutor YouTube Channel:
http://goo.gl/mcbJY

Author
Rob Theriault BHSc., EMCA, RCT(Adv.), CCP(F)

© Copyright 2015, 2010, 2002, 2000
Reproduction of any part of this material, written, audio, visual or electronic, in any form, without the written consent of author is forbidden.

Book cover by: Rick Trombley
Heart illustration by: Catherine Townend

A special thanks to Michelle Cleland who graciously shared a number of her ECGs to help me produce this book.

Table of Content

Introduction 2
Acute Myocardial Infarction 2
Benefits of the prehospital 12 Lead ECG 3
Scene time for 12 Lead ECG acquisition 5
Coronary anatomy 6
Review of complexes, segments and intervals 8
What are the Leads and what do they see? 9
Lead placement 11
Voltage vs Time 17
Step by Step approach to the 12 Lead 18
Focused assessment 19
Signs of infarction 20
Assessment and Management of AMI 26
Hypertrophy 28
Bundle Branch Blocks 32
VT versus SVT with aberrancy 36
Exercises 39
The great impostors 49

Appendix: Vector/Axis estimation 52
About the author 58

Introduction

This workbook is designed for those who wish to learn how to interpret 12-15 Lead ECGs in the acute care setting. It was originally written for paramedics but it is also equally suitable for other health professionals who work in the acute care setting. Because it is a workbook, it is most suited for the classroom or as a supplement for Online education. As the author is a paramedic by profession, this workbook has a decidedly paramedic perspective. However, the interpretation component is generic to all who are tasked with the responsibility of acquiring and interpreting 12-15 Lead ECGs in the acute care setting.

The focus of this workbook is on the recognition of acute myocardial infarction. Several other areas of 12-15 lead ECG which are particularly relevant will also be covered. Pleased take advantage of the QR codes that link to videos and other content/

Acute Myocardial Infarction

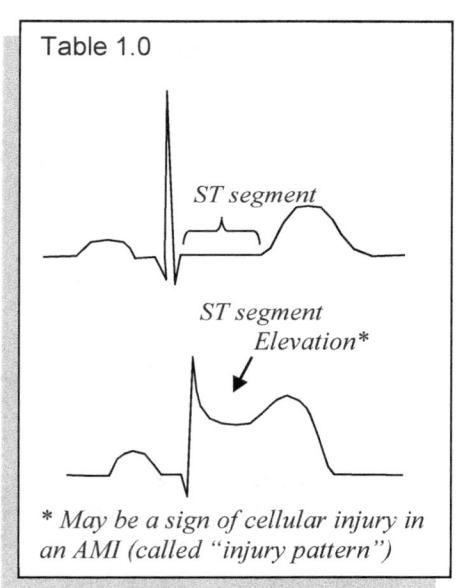

Table 1.0

ST segment

ST segment Elevation*

* May be a sign of cellular injury in an AMI (called "injury pattern")

There are approximately 71,000 heart attacks per year in Canada.[1] In the United States there are 720,000 heart attacks annually[2]. As recently as the 1980s, there was very little that could be done to change the course of myocardial infarction except to provide supportive care and try to prevent sudden death. Myocardial damage would evolve over the ensuing hours and days while health care workers and family watched, waited and hoped. Even today, two thirds of patients who experience an ST segment elevation MI, or STEMI (Table 1.0), will die within the first 24 hours if not treated early[3]. More than half of the deaths occur in the prehospital setting[3].

To address this health crisis, paramedics play a key role in the continuum of care by making a provisional diagnosis of an acute myocardial infarction (AMI) in the field and by initiating treatment. With the advent of thrombolytics, anti-thrombotics and systems allowing paramedics to diagnose AMI and bypass the closest hospital to transport patients to a Percutaneous Coronary Intervention (PCI) Centre, the damage from a myocardial infarction can now be significantly reduced and in some cases reversed. Numerous studies have demonstrated that when paramedics identify ECG changes consistent with an AMI and notify the receiving hospital, this significantly reduces the "door to needle time"[4]. This means that the hospital is able to prepare and to provide reperfusion therapy quicker than they might if they were not notified.

Benefits of the prehospital 12-15 Lead ECG

Chest Pain: Differential diagnosis

As you can see below, the differential diagnosis for AMI is lengthy. Many of the conditions below may have their own distinctive clinical signs or symptoms, however, these conditions may also present with the "classic" symptoms of AMI. Paramedics routinely encounter patients with chest discomfort consistent with cardiac ischemia, and only 10% are having an AMI. For this reason, the 12-15 Lead ECG is an excellent diagnostic tool to narrow the differential diagnosis.

Differential diagnosis
- angina pectoris
- anxiety
- aortic valvular disease or aortic stenosis
- asthma
- cholelithiasis, cholecystitis and biliary colic
- chronic obstructive pulmonary disease and emphysema
- congestive heart failure and pulmonary edema
- endocarditis
- esophagitis
- gastroenteritis
- G.I. bleed
- hypertrophic cardiomyopathy
- mitral valve prolapse/regurgitation
- myocarditis
- pancreatitis
- pericarditis and cardiac tamponade
- pleurisy
- pneumonia
- pneumothorax
- pulmonary embolism
- thoracic aortic dissection
- neoplasm
- thoracic aortic aneurysm, etc

> **Evidence Based Medicine**
>
> The literature suggests that prehospital ECG (PHECG) and advanced notification of the emergency department (ED) reduces in-hospital time to fibrinolysis (thrombolytic treatment).[5]
>
> "It has been conclusively demonstrated that information obtained from the prehospital ECG reduces the time to hospital-based reperfusion treatment. Importantly, these benefits are encountered with little increase in EMS resource use or on-scene time."[6]
>
> Most AMIs occur in persons over the age of forty five[3]. However, younger patients at risk of AMI include cocaine users, patients with insulin-dependent diabetes or hypercholesterolemia, and those with a family history for early coronary disease"[3].

As important as it is to correctly identify STEMI, it is equally important to rule out (R/O) conditions for which, if confused with AMI, the treatment may be lethal – e.g. administration of a thrombolytic in the setting of a thoracic aortic dissection, pericarditis or G.I bleed.

Transportation to the most appropriate hospital

In a number of cities in Canada, paramedic services have adopted a "triage bypass" system whereby when an STEMI has been identified on the cardiogram, the paramedics are authorized to bypass the closest hospital in order to the patient to a "percutaneous coronary intervention" (PCI) Centre.

Differentiating dysrhythmias

VT can seem indistinguishable from SVT with aberrant conduction when the heart rate is high and the P waves are indiscernible. The benefit of the 12 Lead ECG is the ability to look at the heart's electrical activity from 12 or more different perspectives. For example, some leads are better than others at highlighting atrial activity. There are also several other 12 Lead ECG criteria for distinguishing VT from SVT with aberrancy which will be discussed later.

> **Evidence Based Medicine**
>
> One study out of Boston determined that using the prehospital 12 Lead ECG for prehospital triage of suspected STEMI patients will result in the diversion of as many as 22% of patients to hospitals with PCI capability[7].
>
> "AMI patients with prehospital, partial dose thrombolysis followed by immediate transport to a Level I cardiovascular centre (bypassing the closest hospital if necessary) for facilitated infarct-related artery PCI has the potential to reduce the mortality in ST-elevation AMI patients from 6%-10% to less than 4% which could translate into *saving approximately 500 lives per day* in the United States."[8]

The 12 Lead is valuable in differentiating a number of other dysrhythmias, especially when P waves are unclear in standard monitoring leads or when there is excess artefact in some leads but not in others.

Meaningful patient follow up

Most paramedics in Canada are trained in 12 Lead ECG acquisition and interpretation. One of the benefits of learning this interpretation skill is to obtain meaning follow-up on the patient by viewing their hospital ECG. This is an important part of continuing medical education as it may confirm or rule out the paramedic's provisional diagnosis. In addition, for those paramedics who do interpret 12 Lead ECGs, the initial cardiogram is not 100% sensitive for AMI. Consequently, although the patient may be infarcting, the paramedic may not be able to see the ECG evidence until the patient has had a number of serial ECGs in the hospital.

The American Heart Association recommends that paramedics should routinely perform 12 Lead ECGs in patients with cardiac signs and symptoms suspected to be ischemic in origin (Level of evidence: B)[9].

12 Lead acquisition
should not delay transport…

…at least, not excessively

> **Research**
>
> In one study, 12 lead ECG acquisition delayed on-scene time by an average of 3-6 minutes[10]. Nonetheless it was felt that the benefit of the prehospital 12 lead ECG acquisition outweighed any concerns about scene delay.

Coronary Anatomy

There are 2 coronary arteries that come off the base of the aorta: The Right Coronary Artery and the Left Main Coronary Artery

R.C.A.

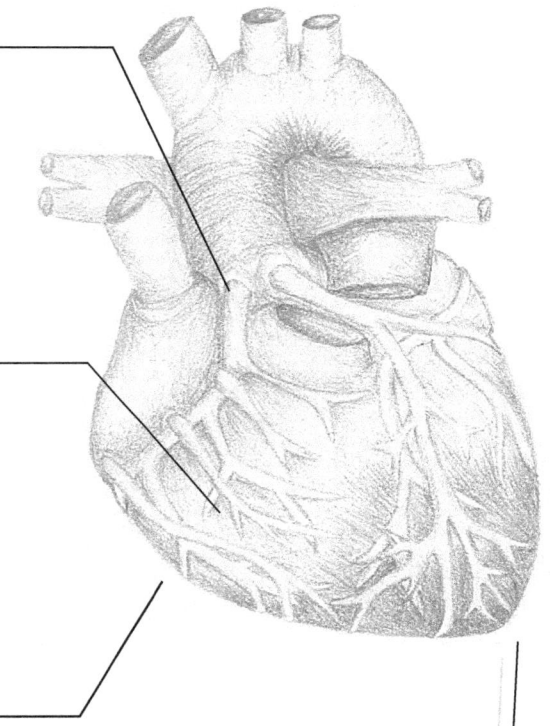

Right Coronary Artery (RCA) comes off the base of the aorta.
It then travels between the right atrium and right ventricle in a groove called the AV sulcus

The RCA feeds:
- ☐ the right ventricle (RV)
- ☐ travels around to the back of the heart, feeding the posterior wall.
- ☐ The RCA also feeds the *inferior wall of the left ventricle* in most humans

Finally, the RCA feeds the SA node in most humans and the AV node in 90% of the population.

Occlusion of the RCA results in infarction of the inferior left ventricle
(ST elevation in Leads II, III, aVF)

Whenever you identify a patient with an inferior wall MI, always look for evidence of a
- posterior wall infarction (ST depression V1-2, ST elevation V7-9
- right ventricular infarct (you have to place right sided precordial leads)

Anticipate
- right ventricular dysfunction and the possibility of hypotension

Coronary Anatomy

Important Coronary Arteries

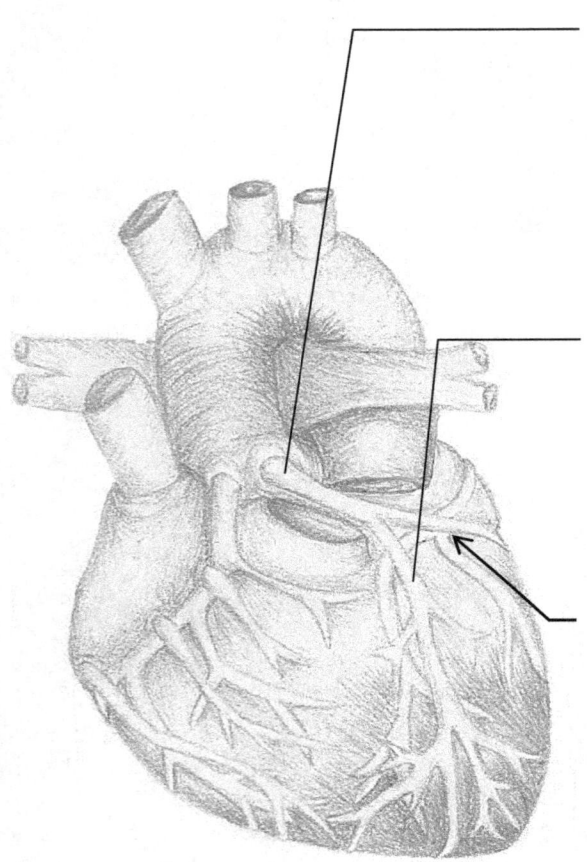

The LEFT MAIN CORONARY ARTERY branches off the base of the aorta and divides into the:
- the *Left Anterior Descending* coronary artery – or the LAD
- the *Left Circumflex* artery (CX)

the LAD supplies blood to the anteroseptal left ventricle
(ST elevation in Leads V1, V2, V3, V4)

The Circumflex Artery travels along the AV sulcus. It supplies blood to the lateral and the posterior left ventricle.
(ST elevation in Leads I, aVL, V5, V6)

- in a small percentage of the population the circumflex supplies the inferior wall of the left ventricle - ST elevation in Leads II, III, aVF, I, aVL, V5, V6,
- i.e. inferolateral MIs

Review of ECG
Complexes, Segments and Intervals

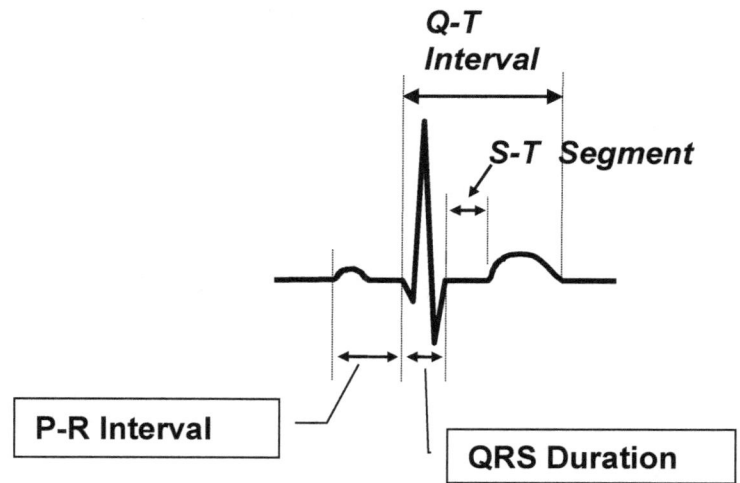

P-R Interval: _____

QRS: _____

ST segment: _____

QT: _____

Normal Q-T

Prolonged Q-T

Prehospital 12 Lead ECG
What are the Leads? What do they see?

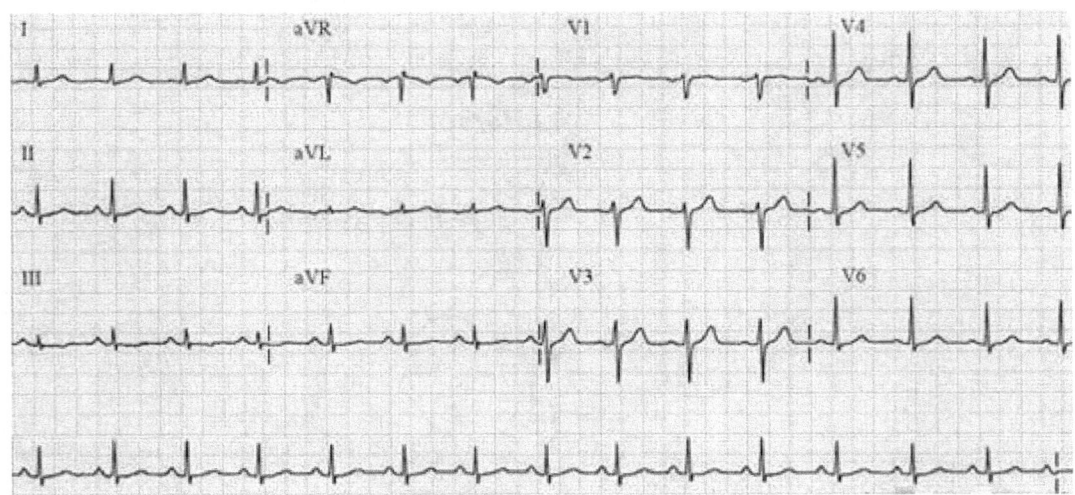

12 different views of the heart

Is the QRS is *typically* positively deflected, negatively deflected of biphasic?:

Lead I: +ve

Lead II: +ve

Lead III: +ve

Lead aVR: -ve *The P wave and QRS are typically negatively deflected. If they're not, Then the leads may be improperly placed*

Lead aVL: +ve

Lead aVF: +ve

Lead V1:   *-ve there is typically a small R wave that represents depolarization of the Intraventricular septum from left to right*

Lead V2:   *mostly -ve*

Lead V3:   *biphasic or equaphasic*   ⎫
Lead V4:   *mostly +ve*   ⎭ *"transition zone"*

Lead V5:   +ve

Lead V6:   +ve

The ECG patterns (P, QRS, ST segment, T) change as a result of ischemia, injury, infarction, electrolyte imbalance, drug toxicity, conduction disturbance, etc

Key Points

- Treat the patient – NOT the ECG

- the 12 Lead ECG is just one more diagnostic tool

- a 12 Lead ECG should be done all patients with chest pain, shortness of breath, dyspnea, or any patient in whom you suspect the potential for altered cardiac function. Also recommended for syncope.

- 15-20% of AMIs have no ECG evidence of infarction – i.e. the 12 Lead ECG has an approximate 80-85% sensitivity for AMI

- When a patient has ECG changes consistent with AMI accompanied by symptoms consistent with cardiac ischemia, the 12 Lead has an almost 100% specificity (accuracy)

- Conversely, there are ECG changes that may masquerade as AMI – to be discussed later.

12-15 Lead Placement

Limb Leads
- Three bipolar leads: I, II, III - measure electrical forces between two leads
- Three unipolar leads: aVR, aVL, aVF ("aV" = augmented vector)
- Six precordial leads (also unipolar)

Limb lead placement

- RA lead: right forearm or wrist
- LA Lead: left forearm or wrist
- LL Lead: left lower leg
- RL Lead: ground lead on the right lower leg

Precordial Leads

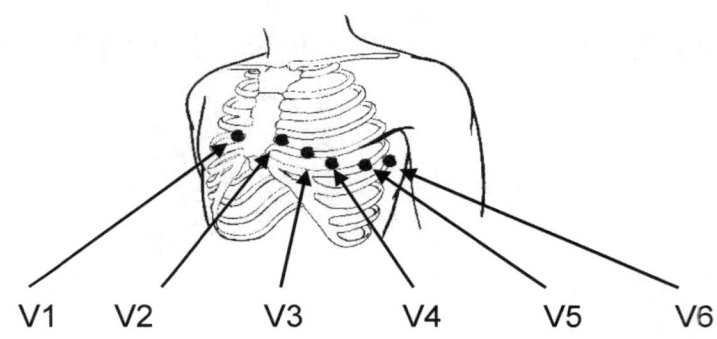

6 Precordial Leads: Horizontal plane leads

VI: 4th intercostal space, right sternal border
V2:   4th intercostal space, left sternal border
V3:   between V2 and V4
V4:   5th intercostal space, mid-clavicular line
V5:   anterior axillary line, in straight line with V4
V6:   mid-axillary line, in straight line with V5

Additional Leads: Right sided precordial leads (15 Lead ECG)
V4R: opposite V4 on the right side of the chest
V5R: opposite V5 on the right side of the chest
V6R: opposite V6 on the right side of the chest

Posterior Leads (if you suspect a posterior wall AMI)
V7: in line with V6 at the posterior axillary line
V8: in line with V6 at the mid-scapular line
V9: in line with V6 at the vertebral border

What Electrodes See

Think of each electrodes as an EYE looking at the heart

Wave of depolarization

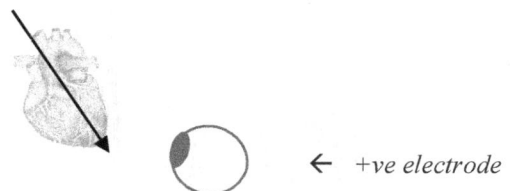

← *+ve electrode*

- When a wave of depolarization moves toward a *+ve* electrode, there will be a positively deflected QRS (**barring any pathology – e.g. old MI**)

- When a wave of depolarization moves away from a +ve electrode, there will be a negatively deflected QRS (e.g. V1, V2, aVR)

- V3 and V4 are referred to as the transition zone

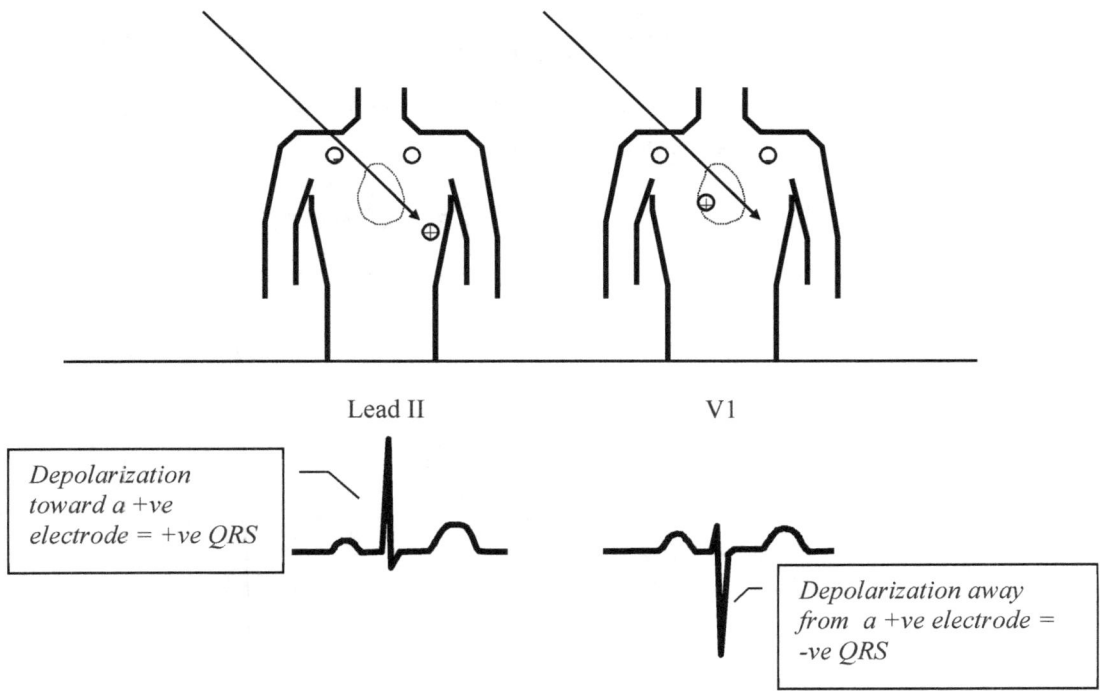

p.12

What Electrodes See

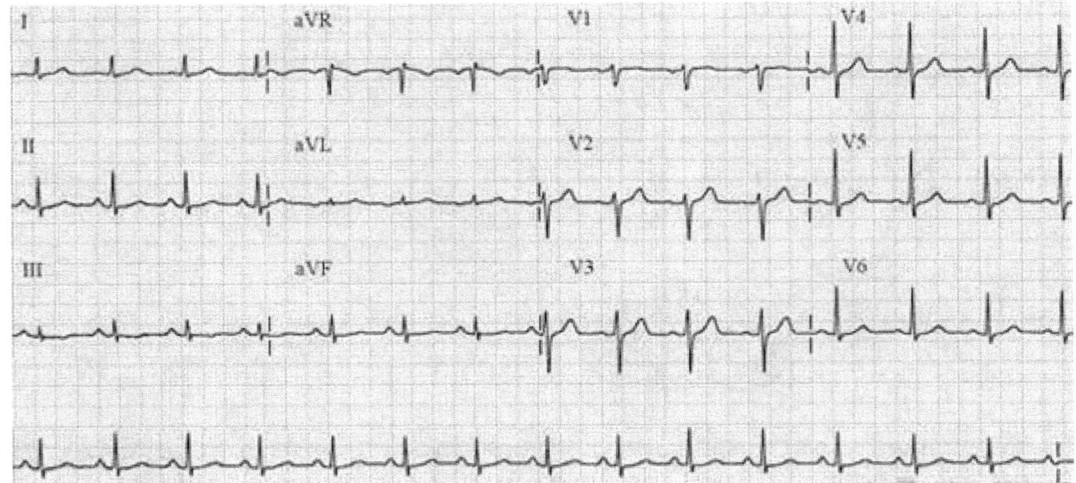

I Lateral left ventricle	aVR	V1 Septal (posterior)	V4 Anterior
II Inferior portion of the heart	aVL Lateral left ventricle	V2 Septal (posterior)	V5 Lateral left ventricle
III Inferior portion of the heart	aVF Inferior portion of the heart	V3 Anterior	V6 Lateral left ventricle
RHYTHM STRIP (not on all 12 Leads)			

Inferior Leads (inferior left ventricle)

I Lateral left ventricle	aVR	V1 Septal	V4 Anterior
II Inferior portion of the heart	aVL Lateral left ventricle	V2 Septal	V5 Lateral left ventricle
III Inferior portion of the heart	aVF Inferior portion of the heart	V3 Anterior	V6 Lateral left ventricle

Which artery supplies the inferior wall of the left ventricle in most humans? (choose one) _____ (RCA / LAD / CX)

If this vessel is occluded, what other parts of the heart should we be clinically concerned about (choose two)? _____
(R. atrium / L. atrium / R. ventricle / L. ventricle / posterior left ventricle)

Anterior Leads - or Anteroseptal Leads (anterior left ventricle)

I Lateral left ventricle	aVR	V1 Septal	V4 Anterior
II Inferior portion of the heart	aVL Lateral left ventricle	V2 Septal	V5 Lateral left ventricle
III Inferior portion of the heart	aVF Inferior portion of the heart	V3 Anterior	V6 Lateral left ventricle

Which artery supplies the anterior or anteroseptal wall of the left ventricle? (choose one) _____ (RCA / LAD / CX)

Left Lateral Leads

I Lateral left ventricle	aVR	V1 Septal	V4 Anterior
II Inferior portion of the heart	aVL Lateral left ventricle	V2 Septal	V5 Lateral left ventricle
III Inferior portion of the heart	aVF Inferior portion of the heart	V3 Anterior	V6 Lateral left ventricle

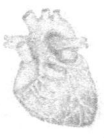

Which artery supplies the lateral wall of the left ventricle? (choose one)
_____ (RCA / LAD / CX)

Anterolateral Leads

I Lateral left ventricle	aVR	V1 Septal	V4 Anterior
II Inferior portion of the heart	aVL Lateral left ventricle	V2 Septal	V5 Lateral left ventricle
III Inferior portion of the heart	aVF Inferior portion of the heart	V3 Anterior	V6 Lateral left ventricle

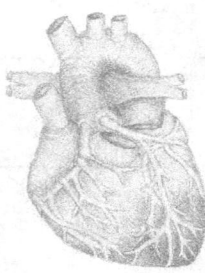

❐ An anterolateral wall infarct results from an occlusion of the left main coronary artery – i.e. before it bifurcates into the LAD and the CX.
❐ This results in a massive infarction! "Acute left main coronary artery obstruction is uncommon and most patients in this clinical setting die of sudden death or cardiogenic shock."[11]

p.15

"Mirror" view of the posterior wall

I Lateral left ventricle	aVR	V1 Septal (posterior)	V4 Anterior
II Inferior portion of the heart	aVL Lateral left ventricle	V2 Septal (posterior)	V5 Lateral left ventricle
III Inferior portion of the heart	aVF Inferior portion of the heart	V3 Anterior	V6 Lateral left ventricle

- When you see a patient with an inferior wall MI (ST ↑ leads I, II, III), **look at leads V1 and V2 for ST segment depression** (mirror image of ST elevation). This change, in the presence of an inferior wall MI, suggests posterior wall involvement or a posterior wall infarction.
- The ST segments are depressed in V1 and V2 because we're looking at a posterior infarct from an anterior perspective.
- To confirm a posterior infarct, run tracings using leads V7, V8 and V9

Lead placement

V7: in a straight line with V6 at the posterior axillary line

V8: in a straight line with V6 and V7 at the mid-scapular line

V9: in a straight line with V6, V7 and V8 at the left vertebral border

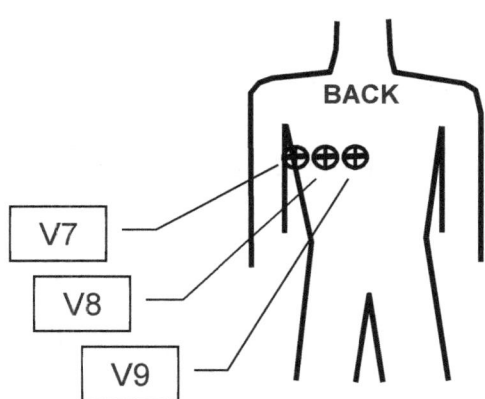

Voltage vs. Time

What the 12-15 Lead ECG really looks at

- When we interpret cardiac rhythms, everything is measured in terms of time on the horizontal axis (e.g. P-R intervals, QRS duration, H.R, etc)

- When we interpret the 12 Lead ECG, we look at voltage which is measured on the vertical axis (e.g. ST segment changes, height of the R wave, depth of the S wave, etc)

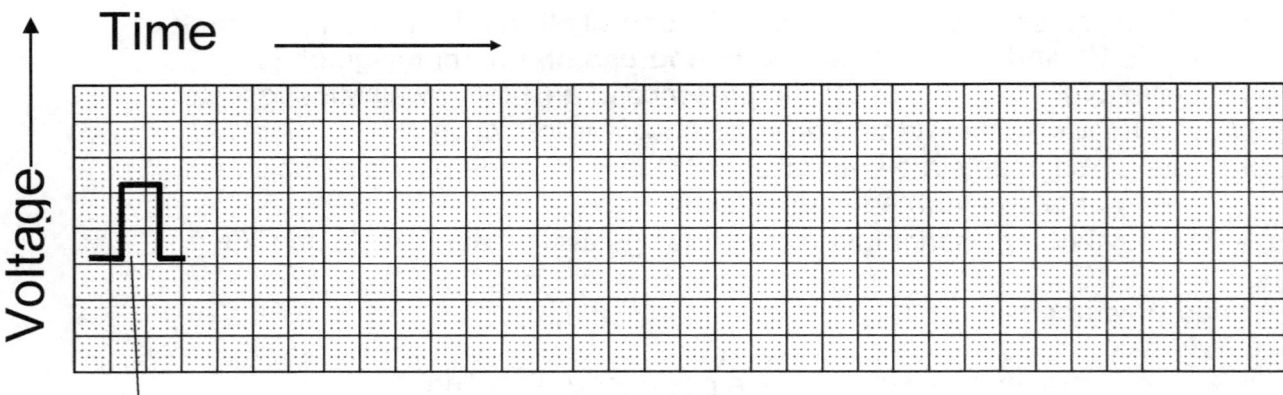

- This deflection is called a "standard"

- You'll see a "standard" deflection on virtually all 12 Lead ECGs

- All 12 Lead ECG machines are calibrated to a "standard" of 1 millivolt (1 mV).

- 1 mV is equal to 1 cm on the graph paper

- If the standard is not 1cm in height then the machine's calibration is off

p.17

Step by Step
12 Lead ECG

- **Rate** (critical information)

- **Rhythm interpretation** (critical information)
    - Intervals
    - Ratio: P to QRS

- **Ischemia, injury and infarction** (critical information)
    - Ask yourself, is the ischemia/injury/infarction due to coronary occlusion or secondary to volume depletion, an excessively fast heart rate, or some other cause?*
    - Which vessel(s) is likely affected? RCA? LAD, CX or left main coronary artery?

- Hypertrophy (for your brain only or FYBO)

- Intraventricular conduction defects (IVCD) - e.g. bundle branch blocks (important or FYBO - use clinical judgement)

- Axis (FYBO)

- Misc.

* What is the heart rate?

- Are the patient's signs and symptoms heart rate related?

- A very slow or excessively fast heart rate may compromise cardiac output and/or coronary blood flow and result in hypotension and/or ischemic chest pain as the heart's metabolic demands exceeds supply

- is there a correctable underlying cause for the slow or fast heart rate?

EXAMPLES

1. reflex tachycardia from volume depletion, anxiety, vasodilator Rx, etc
2. Re-entrant tachyarrhythmias (SVT or VT)
3. Pre-excitation tachyarrhythmias
4. Sinus bradycardia - Treat or not treat?
5. Heart block - treat?

Focused Assessment: Myocardial Infarction

You to the workplace of a 68 y/o male patient, weighing 86 kg, c/o sudden onset of retrosternal chest discomfort he describes as a "squeezing feeling across my chest". He rates it at 4 out of 10 on the pain scale. He is mildly SOB, pale, diaphoretic + and cool to touch. The pain started one hour ago and has not changed and is not affected by position or breathing.

Vitals: HR sinus rhythm of 80 with $\varnothing$ ectopy
RR: 24
B/P: 140/88

O/E: Alert and oriented x3
Neck veins are flat
chest clear with = A/E
Abd: soft, non-distended, non-tender
no peripheral edema noted and PPP x4

Lead II (gives an incomplete picture)

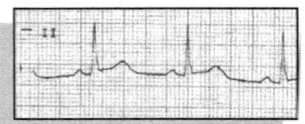

Note that in Lead II there is no ST elevation (i.e. no sign of infarction)

However, when we look at the 12 Lead ECG, we see ST elevation in Leads III and aVF.

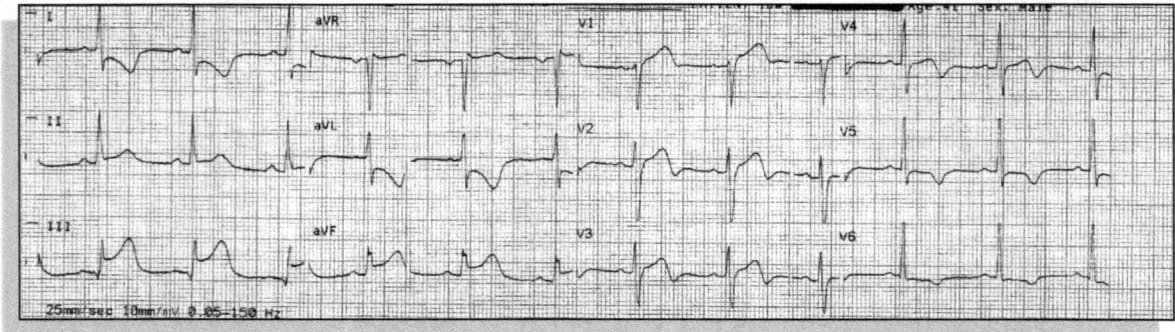

The clinical assessment is critical – The view from a single Lead is inadequate to get the big picture.

Signs of Myocardial Infarction

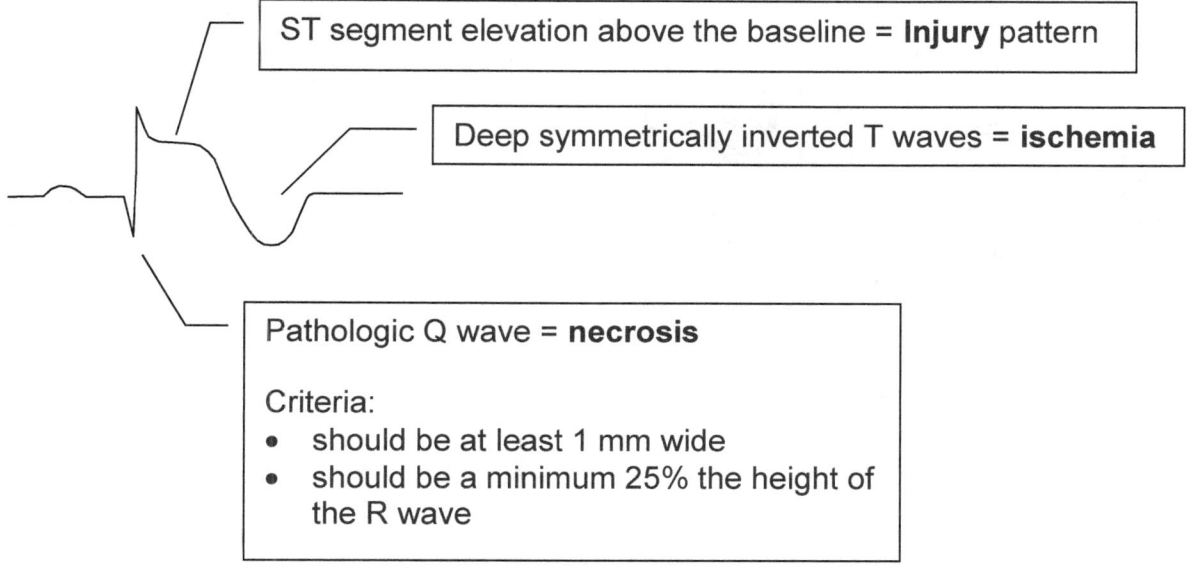

- ST segment elevation above the baseline = **Injury** pattern
- Deep symmetrically inverted T waves = **ischemia**
- Pathologic Q wave = **necrosis**

  Criteria:
  - should be at least 1 mm wide
  - should be a minimum 25% the height of the R wave

- Myocardial infarction is an evolving process
- A coronary vessel suddenly becomes occluded or virtually-occluded and the blood supply becomes inadequate to meet the heart's metabolic demands
- Collateral circulation may help slow the process or limit the size
- **Ischemia** occurs when the blood flow to myocardial tissue becomes inadequate resulting in tissue hypoxia.
- Some cells may become "injured" (common initial ST ↑ pattern in AMI)
- **Injury** occurs as a result of severe ischemia and alters cell membrane function – this is ST elevation MI or **STEMI**
- **Infarction** is defined as tissue death from inadequate blood and/or oxygen supply.

- *In an acute myocardial infarction, you may not see all three changes – see example below.*

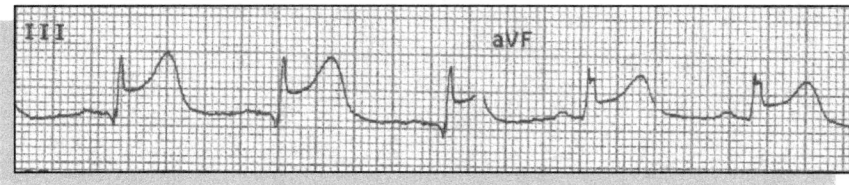

Note in this acute MI that we only see ST elevation – no inverted T waves or pathological Qs. This is a common ECG pattern in the early phase of AMI

p.20

Sample: Inferior Wall MI

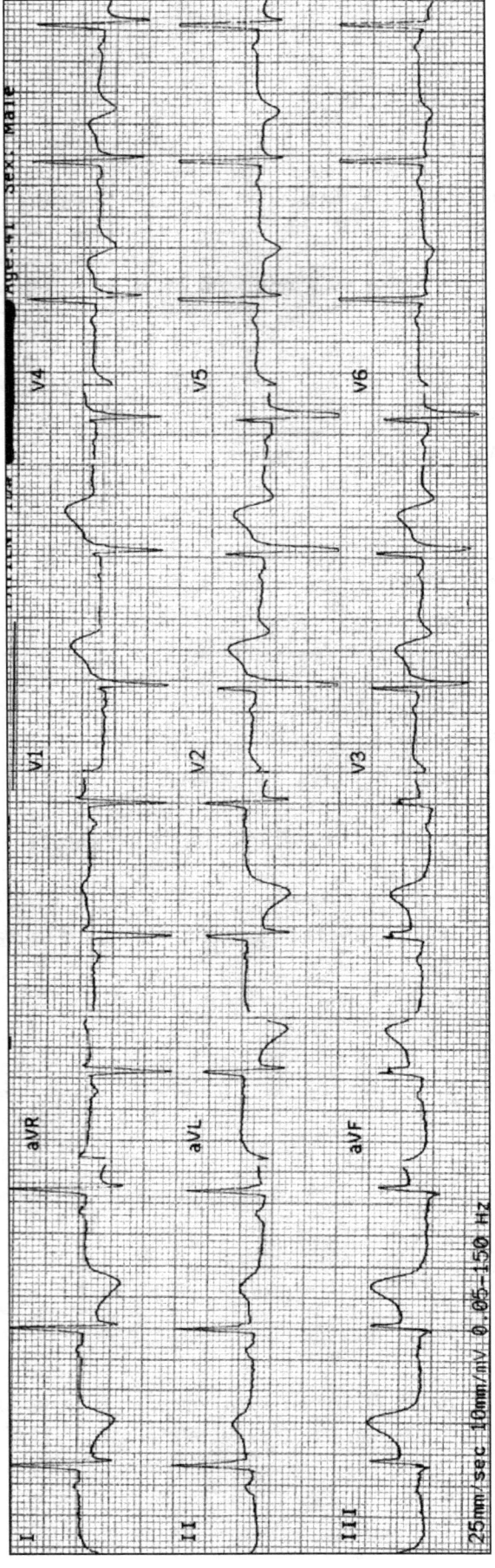

Reciprocal changes
In an AMI you're looking for ST ↑ in two or more contiguous leads. The presence of ST ↓ in other leads may be a sign of reciprocal changes. These are sometimes called mirror images but are simply leads looking at the same infarction from a different angle. Not all AMIs have reciprocal changes, but it's critically important to look for it to confirm it's am MI and not an MI mimic. e.g. In an Inferior wall MI, such as the one above, look for ST ↓ in the lateral leads I, aVL. In anterior or lateral wall MIs look for ST ↓ in II, III, aVF.

p.21

Sample: Right Ventricular Infarction

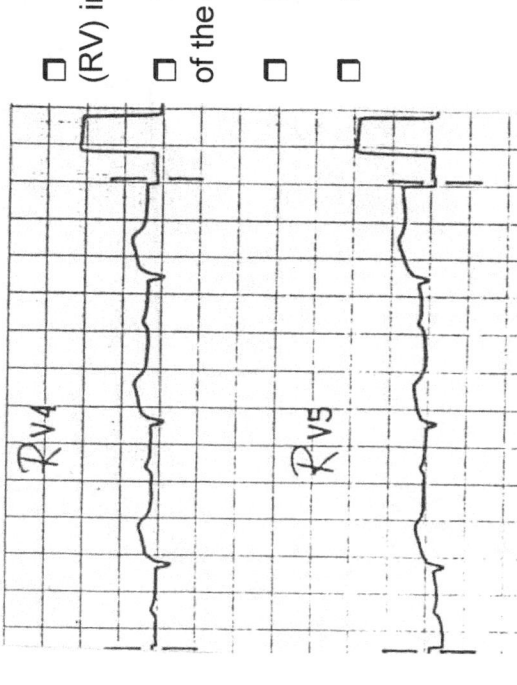

- ☐ In the setting of an inferior wall MI, look for evidence of a right ventricular (RV) infarct - *this is always a concern when you believe the RCA is occluded*
- ☐ RV4-RV6 are placed in the same positions as V4-V6, but on the right side of the chest
- ☐ Run a 12 Lead strip and re-label the leads with an "R"
- ☐ ST elevation in any of these leads is indicative of an RV infarct

Clinical signs of a RV infarct

- ☐ Hypotension (+/- altered LOA)
  - o Potential for *shock*
- ☐ Normal or slow heart rate
- ☐ Chest is clear on auscultation
- ☐ JVD

Clinical caveat
The right ventricle does not contract effectively in the setting of a RV infarct. Since the right ventricle is preload dependant, administering Nitroglycerin, a preload reducer, can have disastrous consequences. Patients frequently respond well to fluid resuscitation.

p.22

Sample: Anterior wall MI

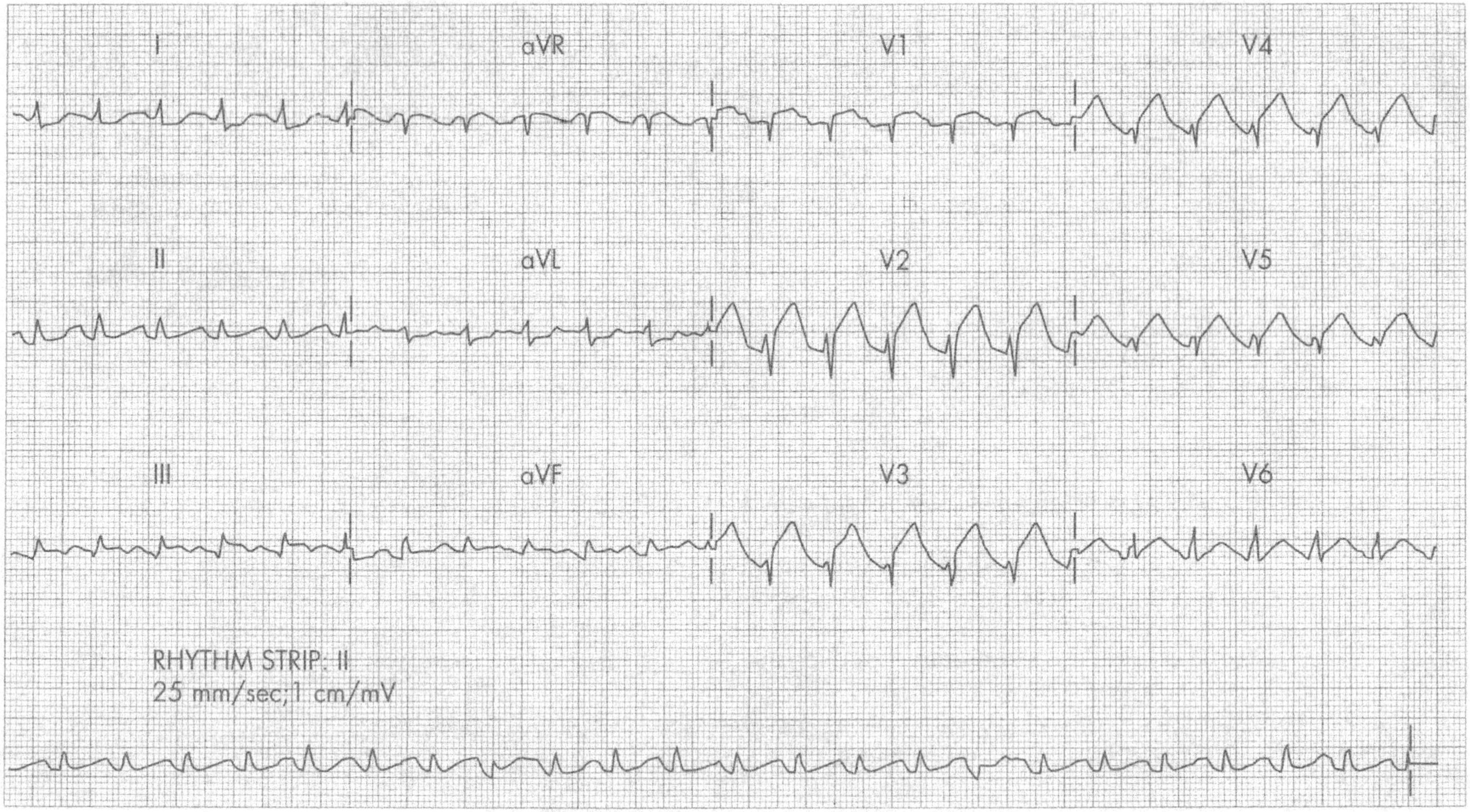

Sample: Evolving MI

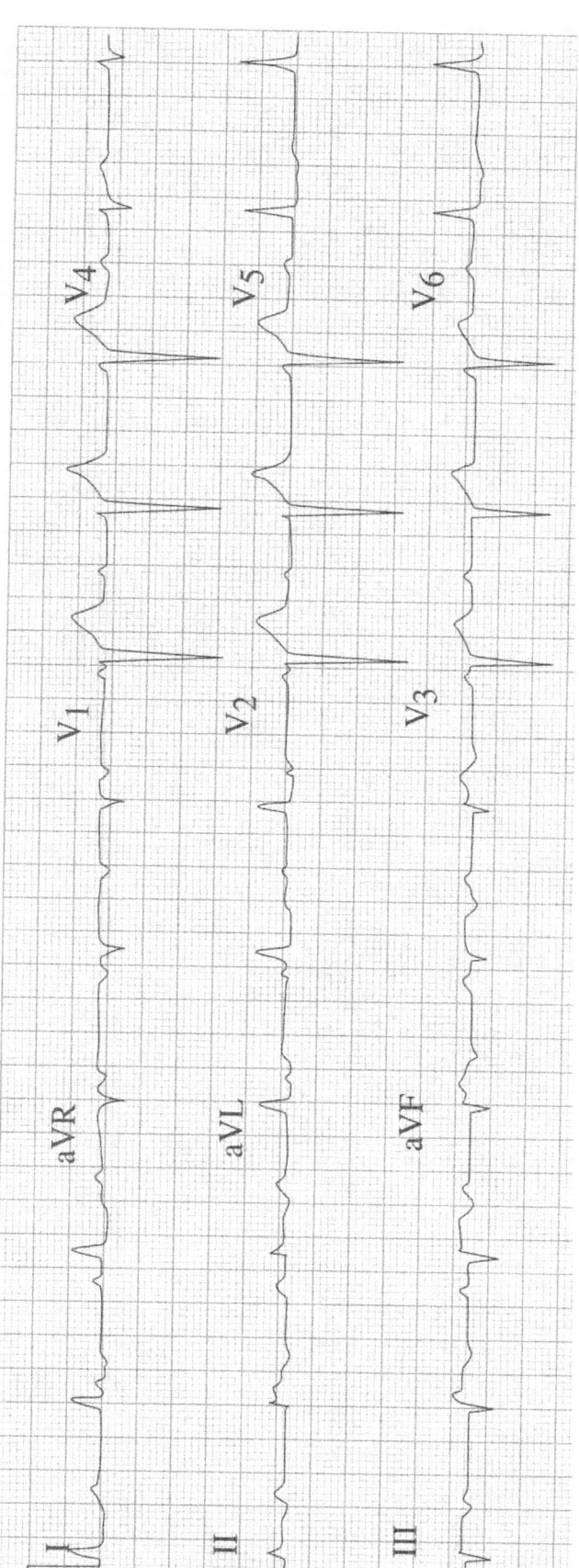

Sample: Old Inferior wall MI

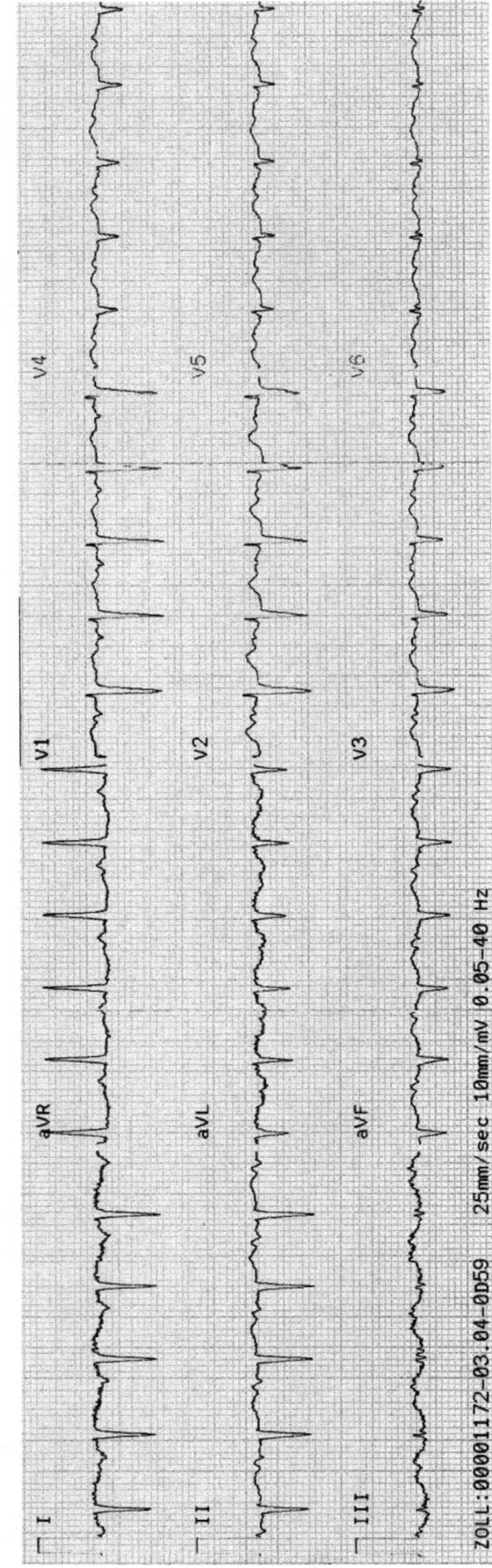

Assessment & Management of AMI

Step 1:
- ABCD, exam, 12-15 Lead ECG – hunt for STEMI, differential diagnosis

Step 2:
- Initiate treatment: Rule out Inferior AMI prior to giving NTG, transport to PCI?

Step 3:
- Transport to PCI Centre (if this is an option)
- Screen for Thrombolytics (important information whether giving it in the field or not)
    - Rule out contraindications
        - active bleeding
        - thoracic aortic aneurysm
        - pericarditis

    - **relative contraindications** to thrombolytic therapy
        - recent surgery, recent trauma, recent stroke, pregnancy, recent GI bleed, prolonged CPR

AMI: Prehospital Treatment Objectives

- problem is one supply and demand
- you can alleviate pain by ↑O_2 and perfusion (supply to the heart) and/or by decreasing MVO_2 (e.g. preload reduction, HR reduction)

1. Position of comfort; sitting - unless pt is hypotensive (reducing demand)

2. FiO_2: Some controversy exist over whether O_2 is beneficial (↑ supply)

3. NTG _____ SL reduces preload (↓ MVO_2) dilates coronary arteries (↓ demand & ↑ supply)

4. ASA, in low dose, inhibits Thromboxane A2 which is a platelet aggregate and vasoconstrictor – ASA is an anti-thrombotic that limits the size of the infarct

5. Morphine _____ mg (or other analgesia) aliquots _____ preload - analgesic ↓ anxiety = ↓ catecholamine release (↓ demand)

6. Nitro infusion _____/min IV and titrate for management of continuous or recurrent pain   (↓ demand & ↑ supply)

Criteria for Transport to PCI Centre

Fundamental Principle: Patients with the largest infarctions will benefit the most from thrombolytic therapy (follow local policy)

- Signs/symptoms consistent with AMI (refer to local policy about time criteria)
- A single ECG showing ST ↑ signifies the need for transport to PCI and/or prehospital fibrinolysis
- fibrinolytic therapy indicated if eligible patient with anticipated time to primary PCI exceeding 90 minutes
- ST elevation ≥ 1mm in 2 or more anatomically contiguous limb leads

OR

- ≥ 2mm (1.5mm in women) in 2 or more anatomically contiguous precordial leads,

OR

- In the presence of LBBB: look for Modified Sgarbossa Criteria (web search)

ST Segment Scoring

- 7 mm or more combined ST elevation in the limb leads (II, III, aVF) signifies an extensive inferior wall MI
- 12 mm or more combined ST elevation in the precordial leads (V1-V6) signifies an extensive MI

STEMI Equivalents:
- Posterior AMI: ST depression in ≥2 precordial leads (V_1–V_4) may indicate transmural posterior injury
- LMCA AMI: ST depression in multiple leads combined with ST ↑ in lead aVR has been described in patients with left main or proximal left anterior descending artery occlusion.

> **Clinical Caveat**
> Once you've confirmed an AMI in the field and you've been cleared to transport directly to a PCI Centre, consider removing the 12 Leads and applying defibrillation pads. The risk of cardiac arrest enroute is low, however the success of defibrillation is time dependent.

Ventricular Hypertrophy
Increased Muscle Mass

- "No muscle works harder, longer or more steadily than the heart"

- When the heart is forced to work harder than it should, it may become enlarged or hypertrophy

Causes
- increased resistance to outflow - e.g. aortic stenosis, chronic hypertension, valvular regurgitation

ECG
- Since voltage is measured on the vertical axis of the ECG and since ventricular enlargement (hypertrophy) results in a greater amount of electrical activity in the affected chamber, you can expect to see larger than normal QRSs

Left Ventricular Hypertrophy

- Axis is shifted to the left (see Appendix A)
- The S in V1 becomes deeper
- The R in V5 and V6 becomes taller

- Many voltage criteria have been proposed
- if the S wave in V1 or V2 is $\geq$ 30 mm deep

or
- if the R wave in V5 or V6 is $\geq$ 30 mm tall, then left ventricular hypertrophy (LVH) exists
- ST segment depression and T wave inversion can occur - especially in the lateral leads (also called: left ventricular strain pattern

Exceptions - where greater than normal voltage occurs in the absence of hypertrophy:

- people with very thin chest wall
- children
- tall athletes - e.g. basketball players

Atrial Hypertrophy

Look at P wave in Lead V1 or MCL 1

Right atrial hypertrophy

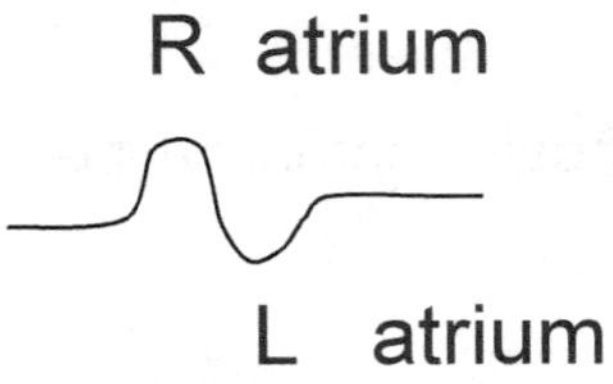

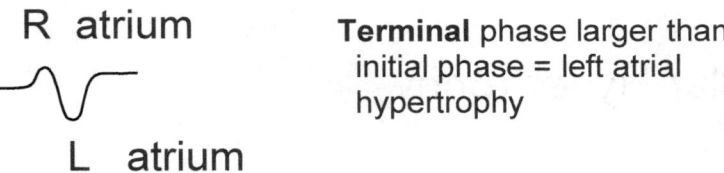

Initial phase larger than terminal phase = right atrial hypertrophy

Left atrial hypertrophy - More common

Terminal phase larger than initial phase = left atrial hypertrophy

Clinical Vignette
Identifying atrial hypertrophy is not important in the field. This purpose of this description is just to provide an understanding that P waves sometimes have a different morphology either due to hypertrophy or because the P was originates from an ectopic site.

Sample: Left ventricular hypertrophy

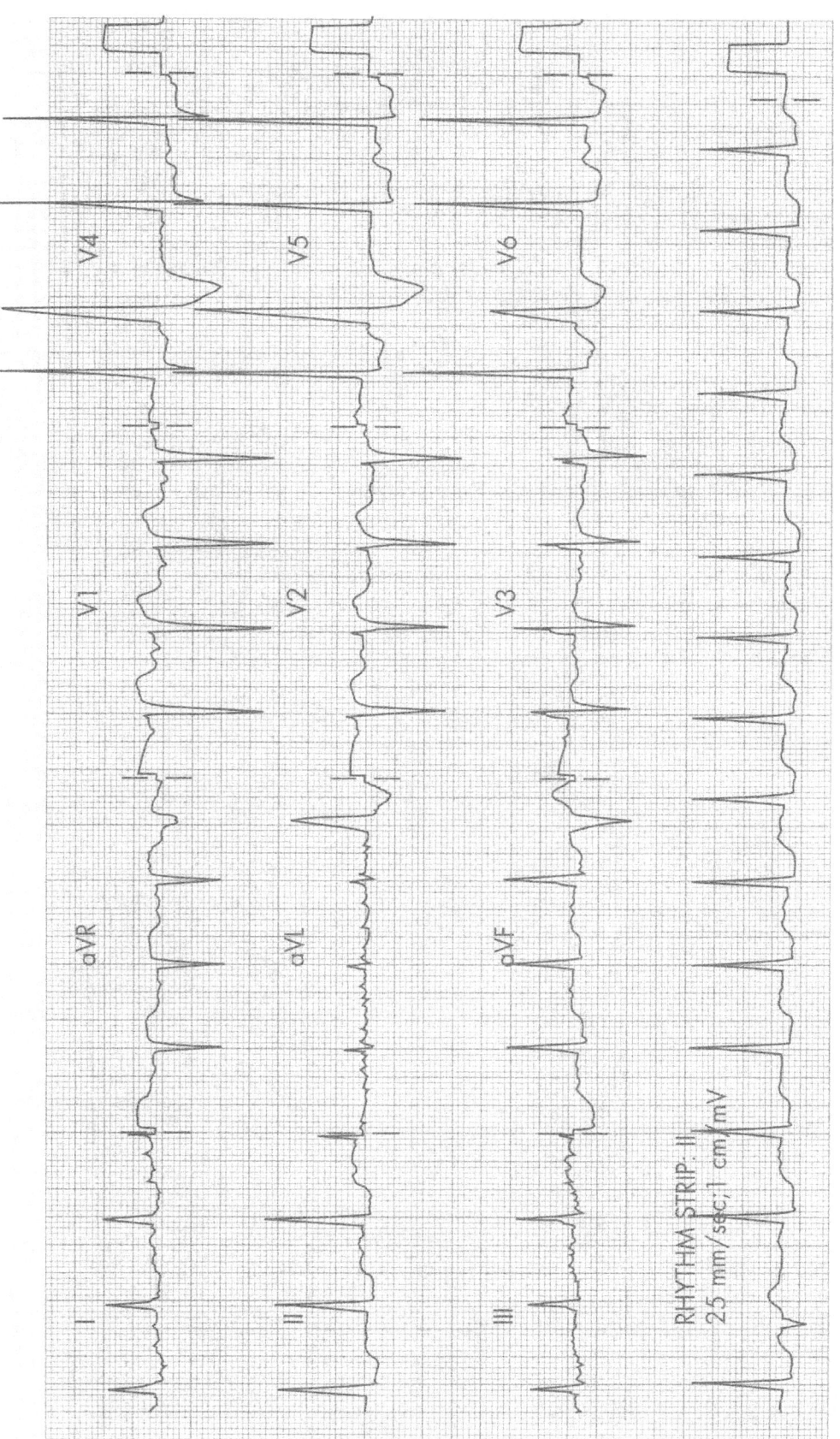

Sample: Atrial hypertrophy

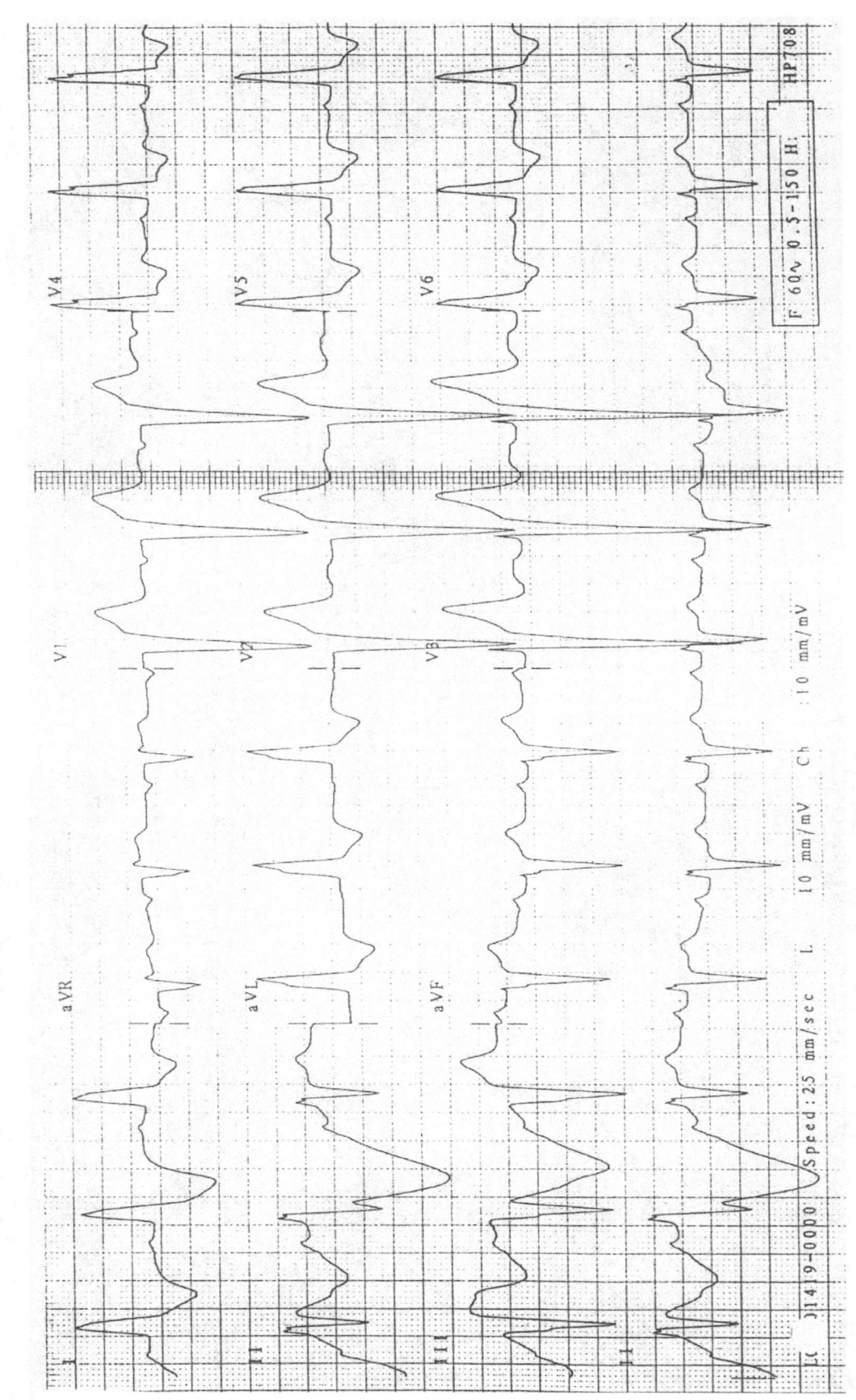

Bundle Branch Blocks

Causes

- MI
- Degenerative disease
- hypoxia
- Electrolyte imbalance
- Rate related
- CHF

Right BBB

- The right Bundle is longer and thinner
- Right bundle is supplied by the Left Anterior Descending coronary artery only
- RBBBs are more common than LBBBs
- V1 and V6 as well as I and aVL are used to diagnose RBBB

Right Bundle Branch Block

- ☐ Wide QRS (P wave preceding each QRS)
- ☐ V1 will show an rSR' (R' = R prime) pattern
- ☐ V1 will be positively deflected - not normal

Lead V1

Lead V6

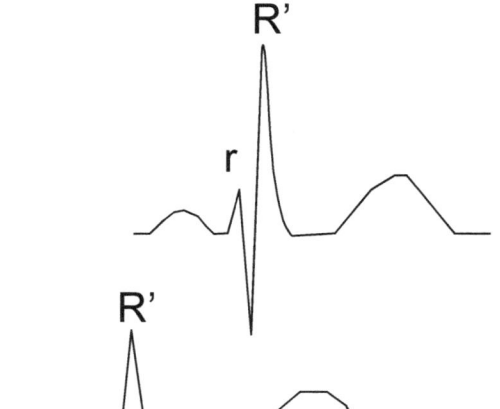

Left Bundle Branch Block (LBBB)

Left BBB

- Wide QRS (P wave preceding each QRS)
- Less common than RBBB
- The left bundle branch is thicker and shorter

V1 will be negatively deflected

Lead V1 will show a QS wave

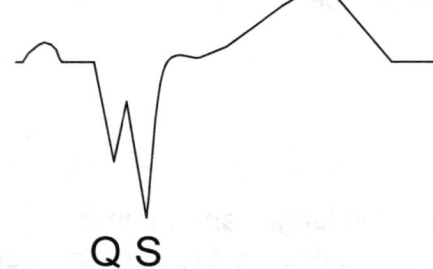

Lead V6, I and aVL

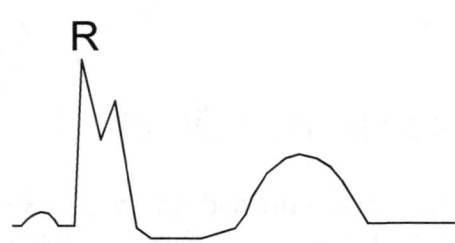

Sample: Right Bundle Branch Block (RBBB)

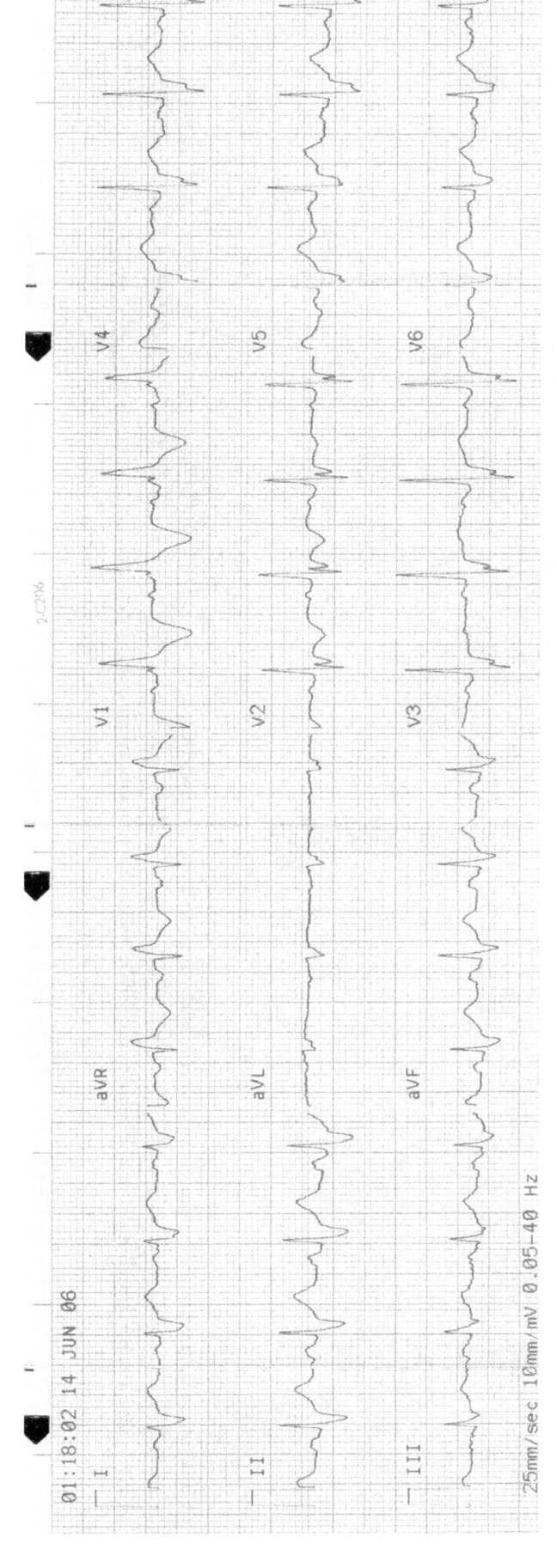

Sample: Left Bundle Branch Block (LBBB)

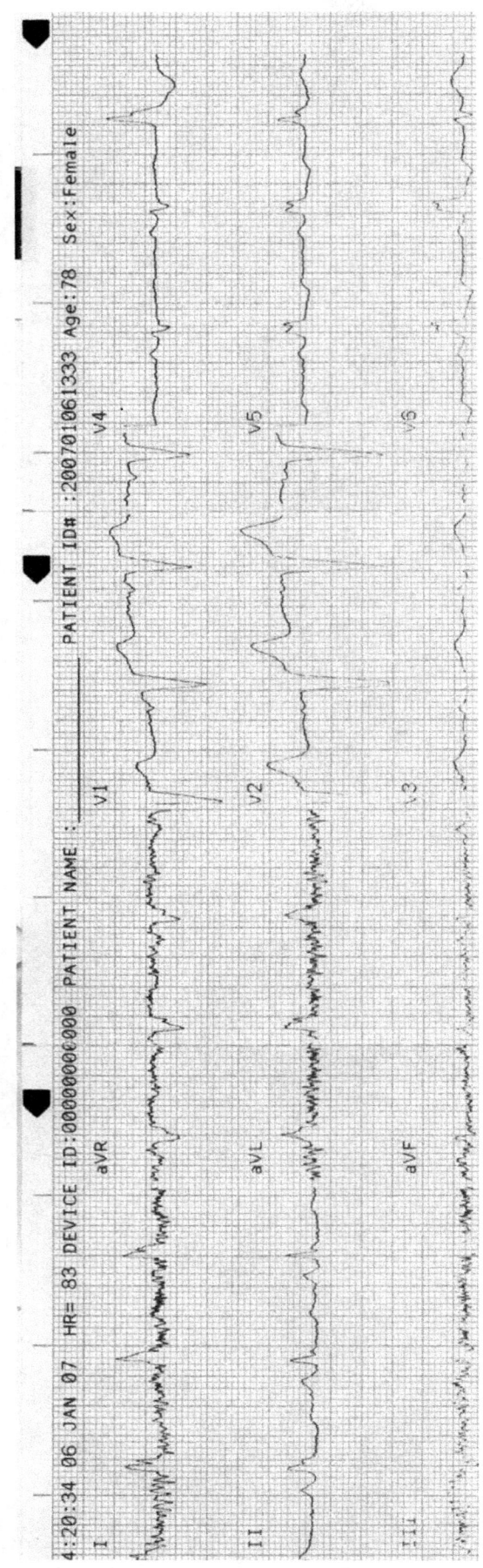

Clinical Vignette

It's difficult to diagnose an AMI when a LBBB is present. This is because in LBBB the right ventricle depolarizes first, hence this is what we're seeing on the electrocardiogram and the usual evidence of left ventricular infarction is absent. Do a web search for Modified Sgarbossa's Criteria.

VT vs. SVT with Aberrancy

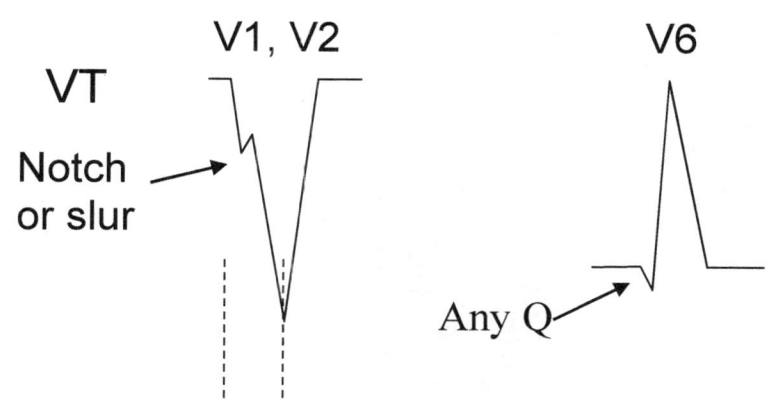

VT
V1, V2 — Notch or slur
V6 — Any Q

Onset of the QRS to the base of the QRS is > 0.06

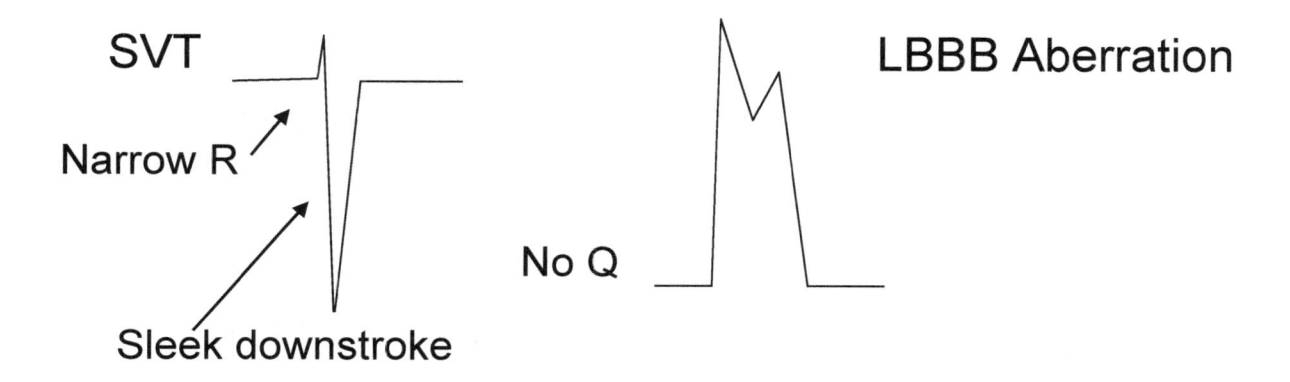

SVT
Narrow R
Sleek downstroke
No Q

LBBB Aberration

Other signs that favour VT

- Uncertainty: i.e. wide complex tachycardia without discernable P waves is a VT until proven otherwise.
- No evidence of bundle branch block pattern
- Concordance: All QRS in V1-V6 are deflected in the same direction
- Extreme right axis deviation: QRS is positive in aVR and negative in I + aVF
- AV dissociation (50%)
    - P waves that "march through"
    - irregular jugular venous distension (as the atria contract against closed AV valves, the blood backs up into the neck)

Sample: Ventricular Tachycardia

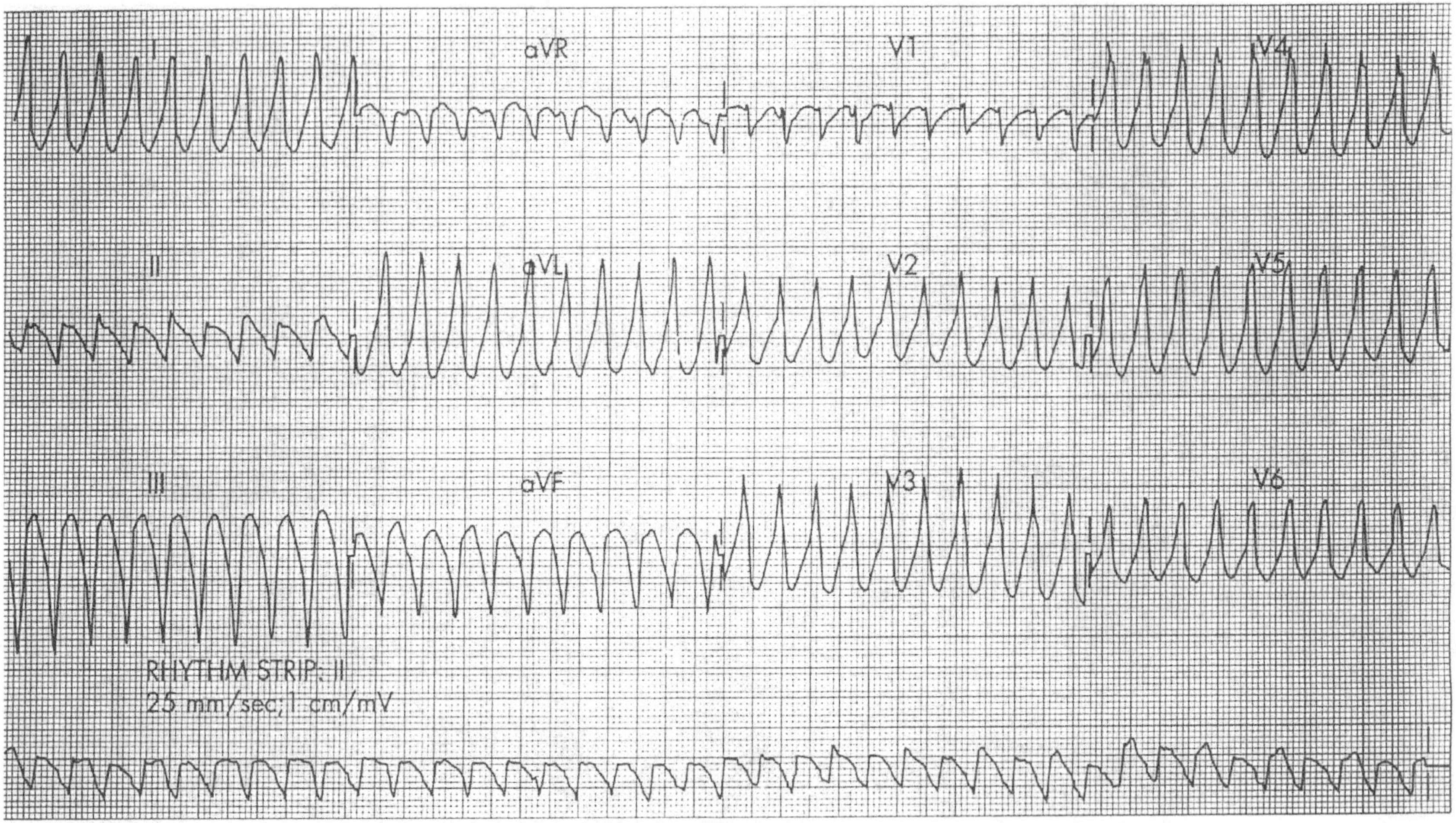

Sample: SVT with aberrancy

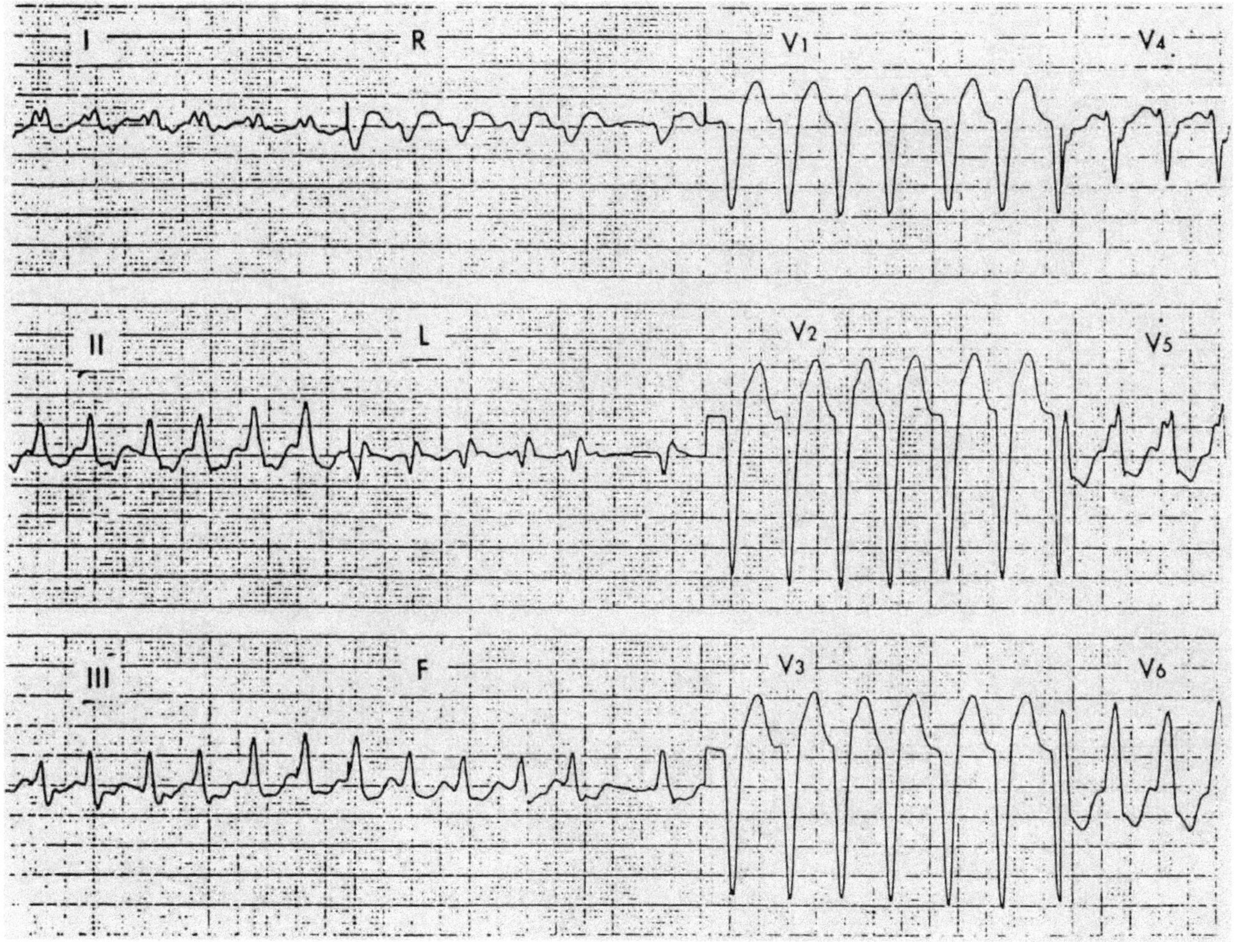

Exercise #1

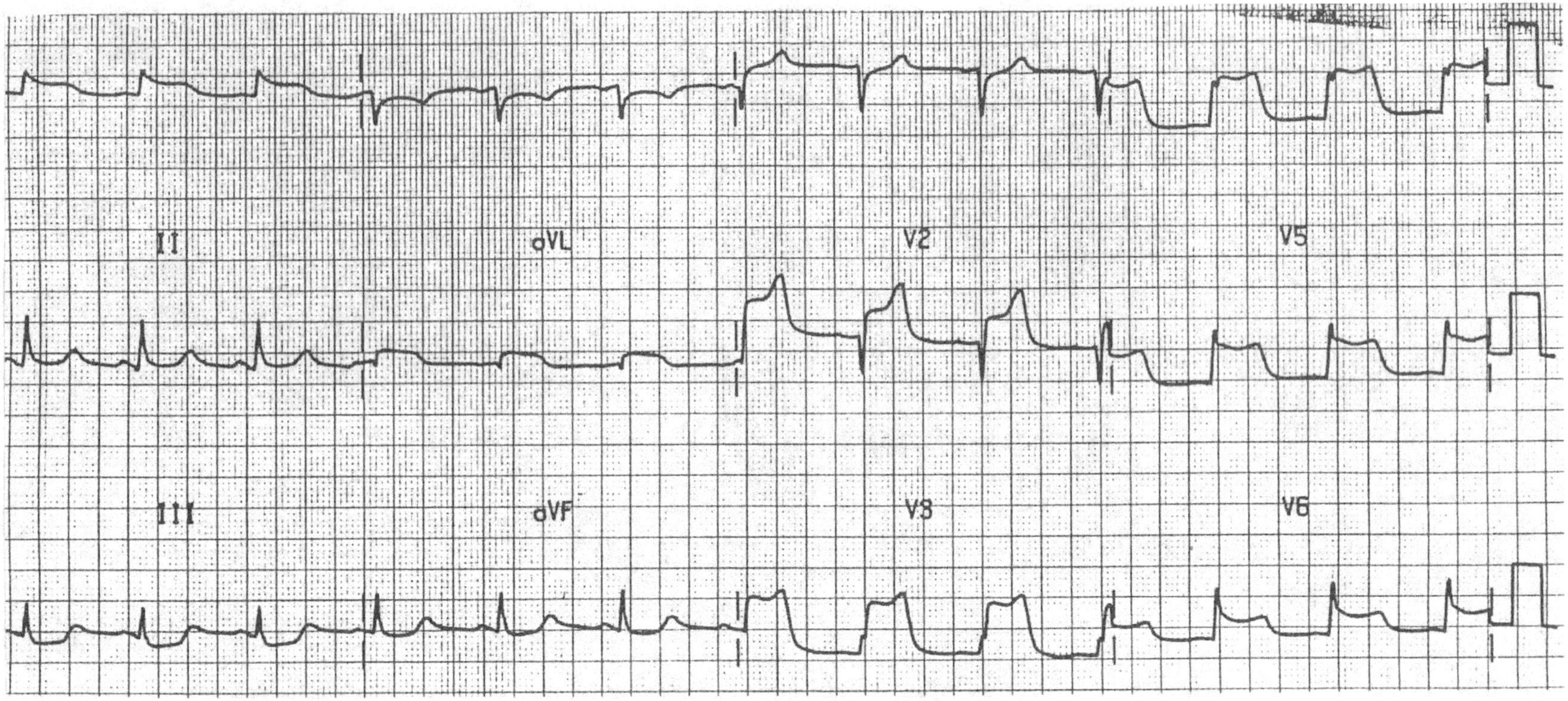

Exercise #2

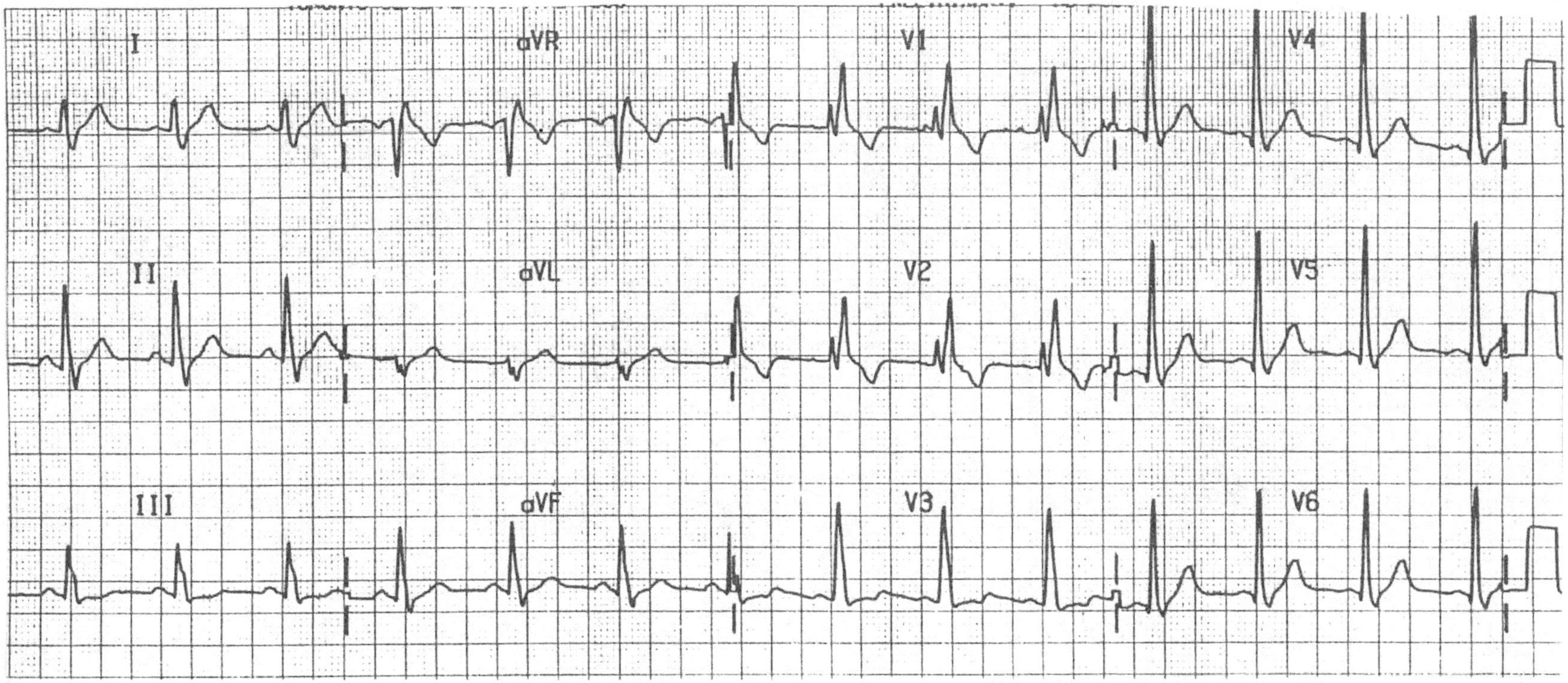

Exercise #3

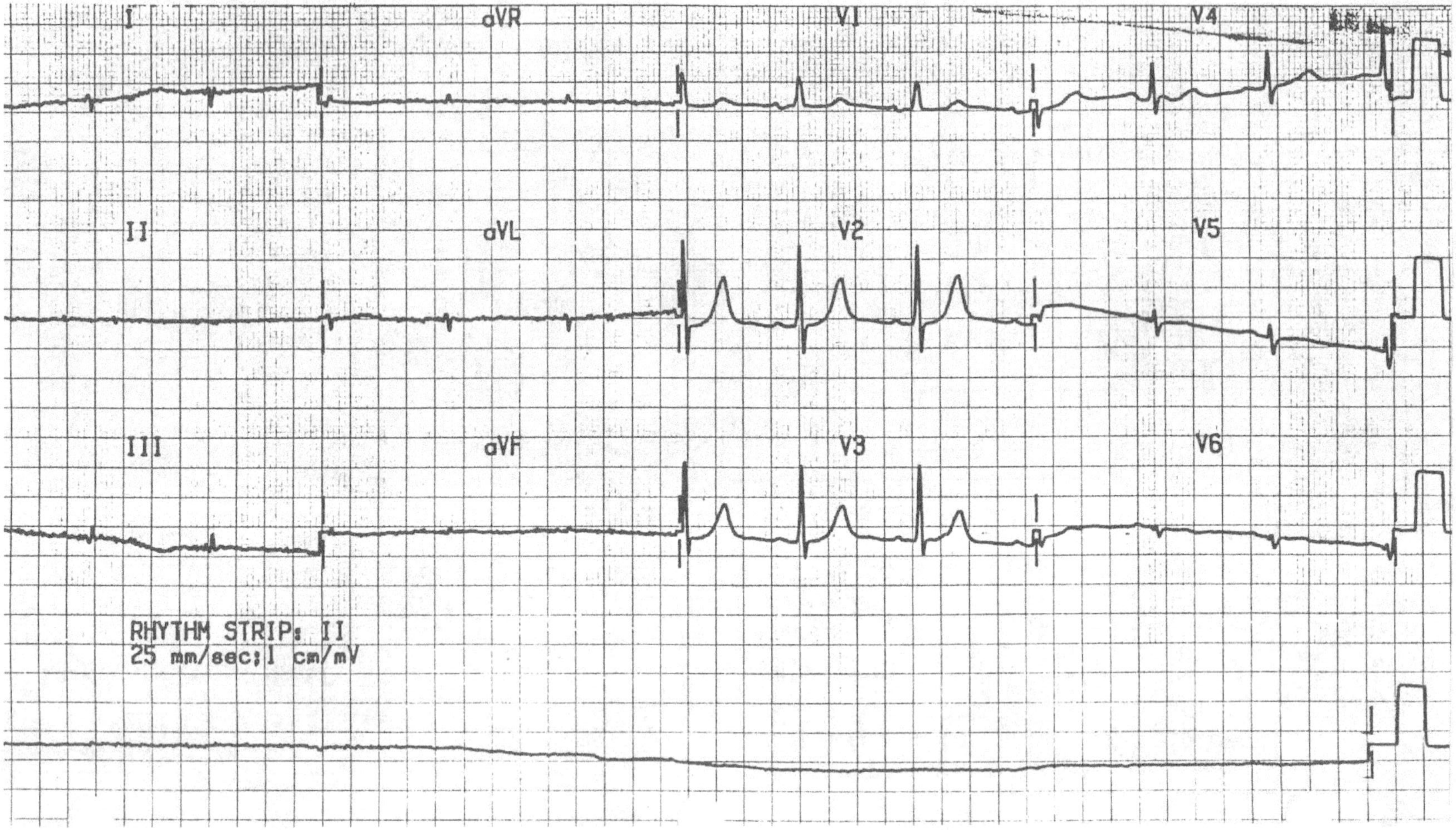

Exercise #4

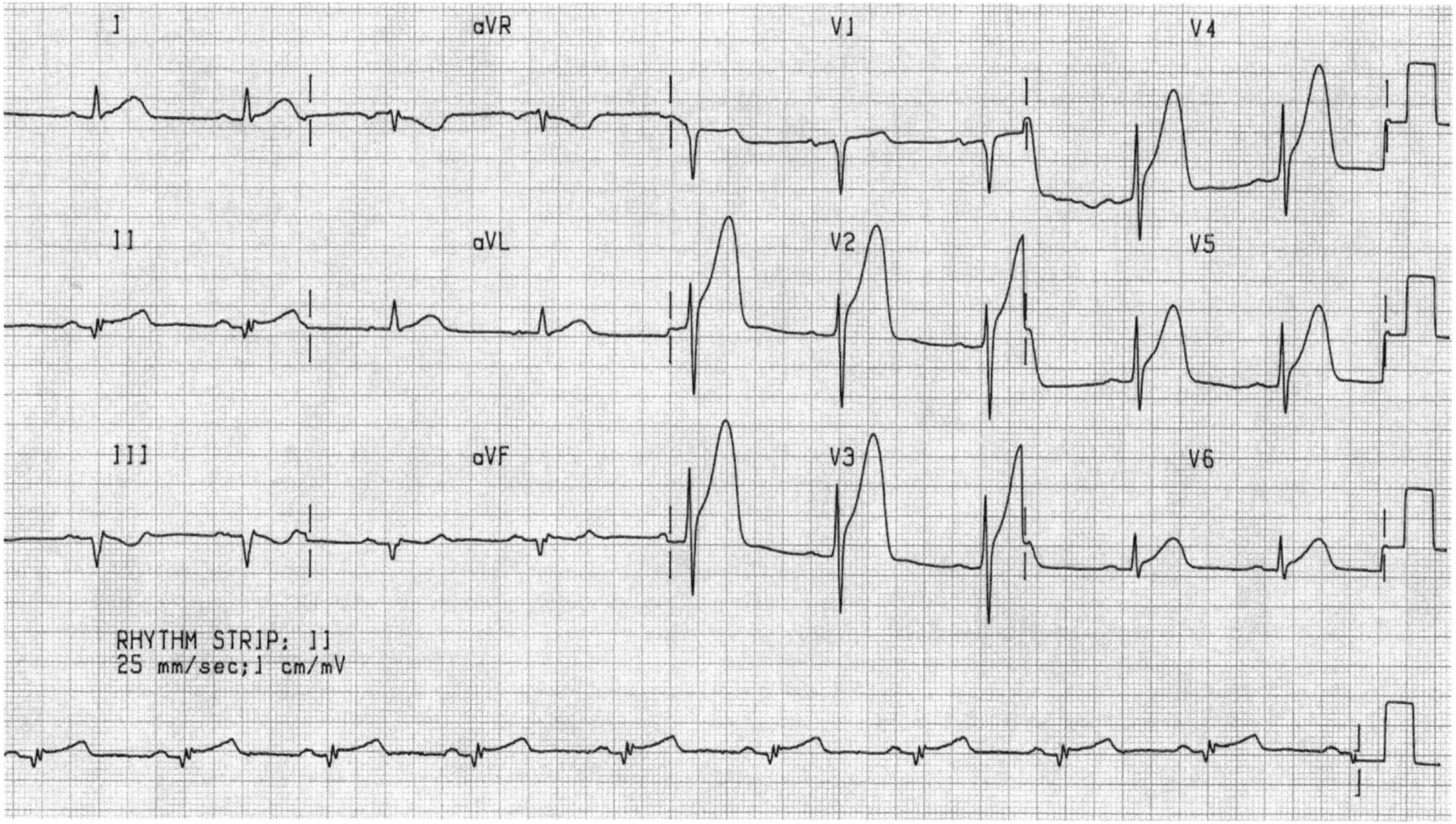

I, II, III, aVR, aVL, aVF, V1, V2, V3, V4, V5, V6

RHYTHM STRIP: II
25 mm/sec; 1 cm/mV

p. 42

Exercise #5

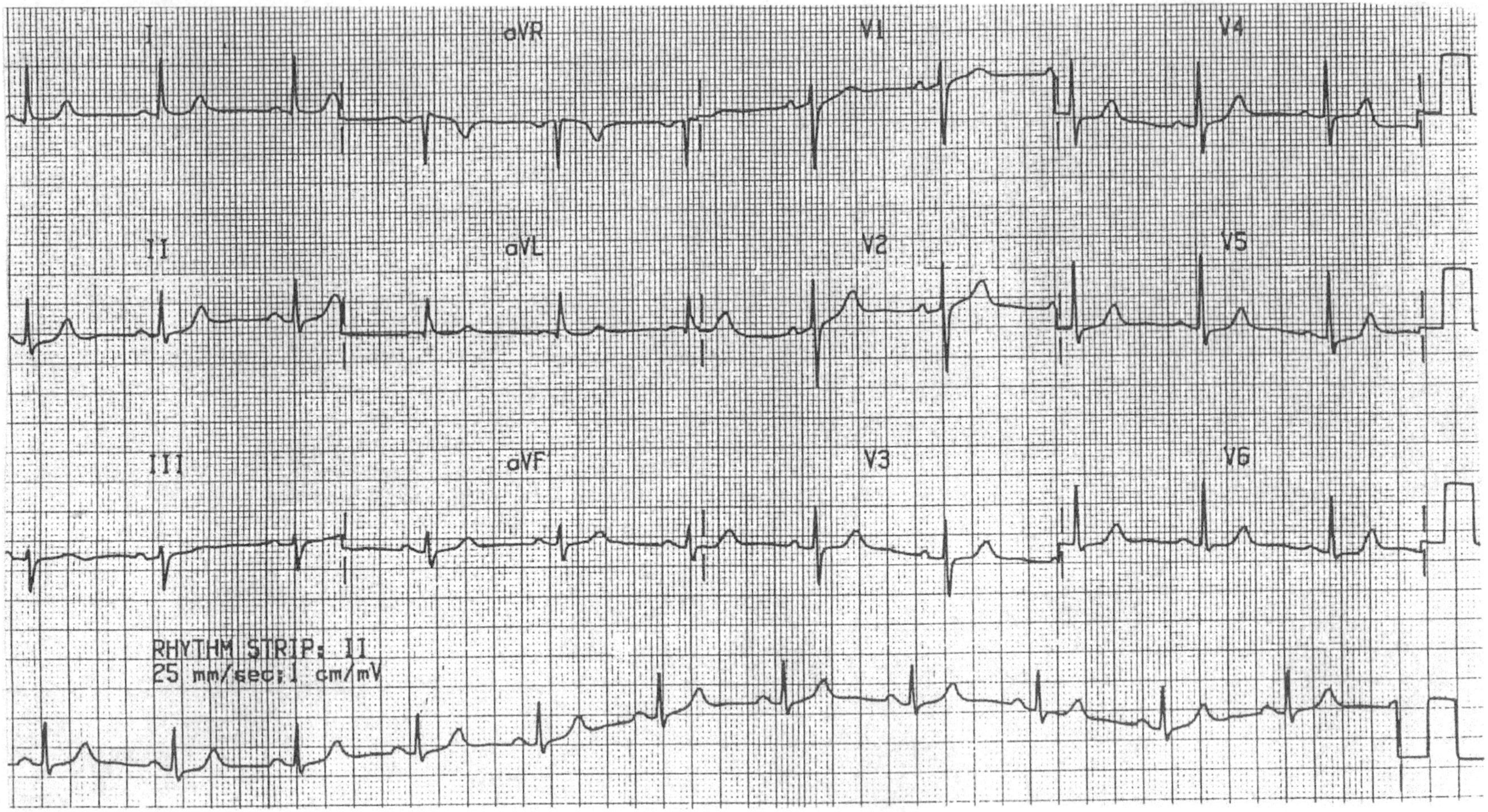

Exercise #6

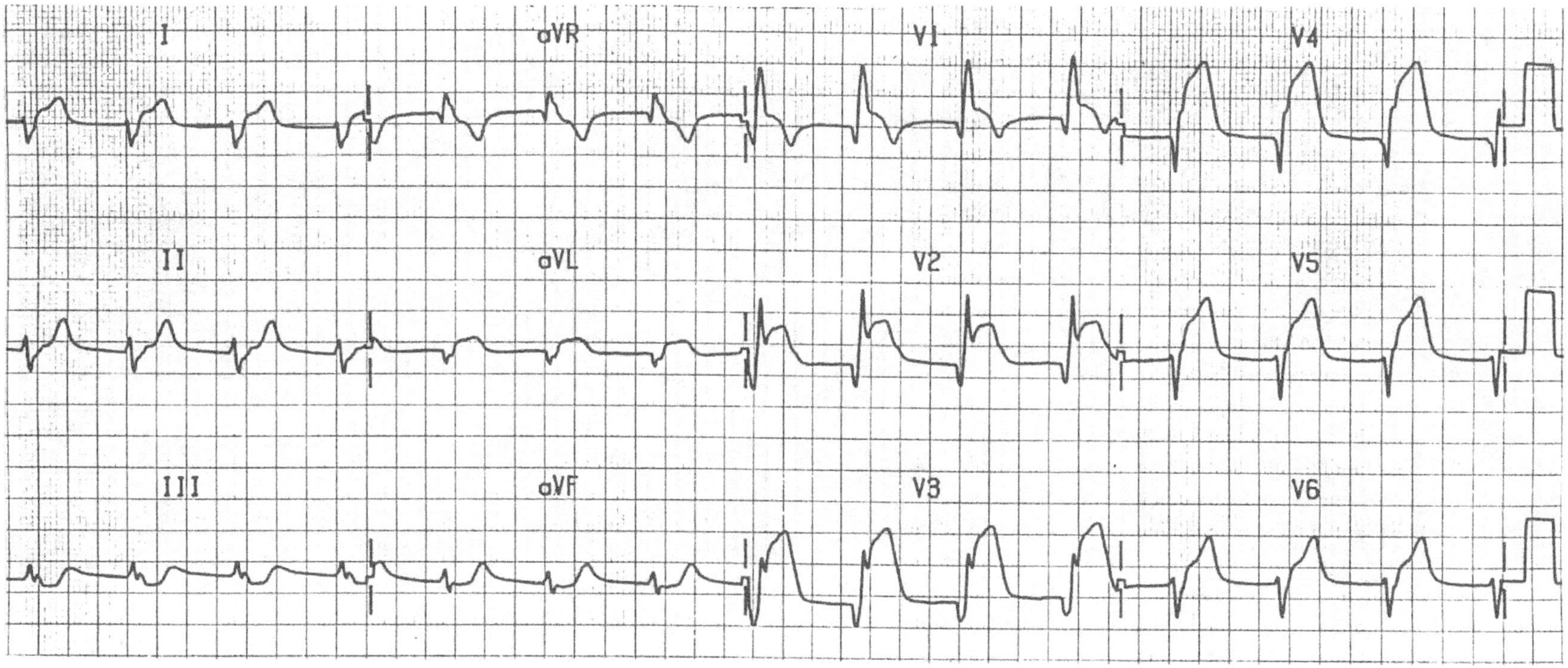

Exercise #7

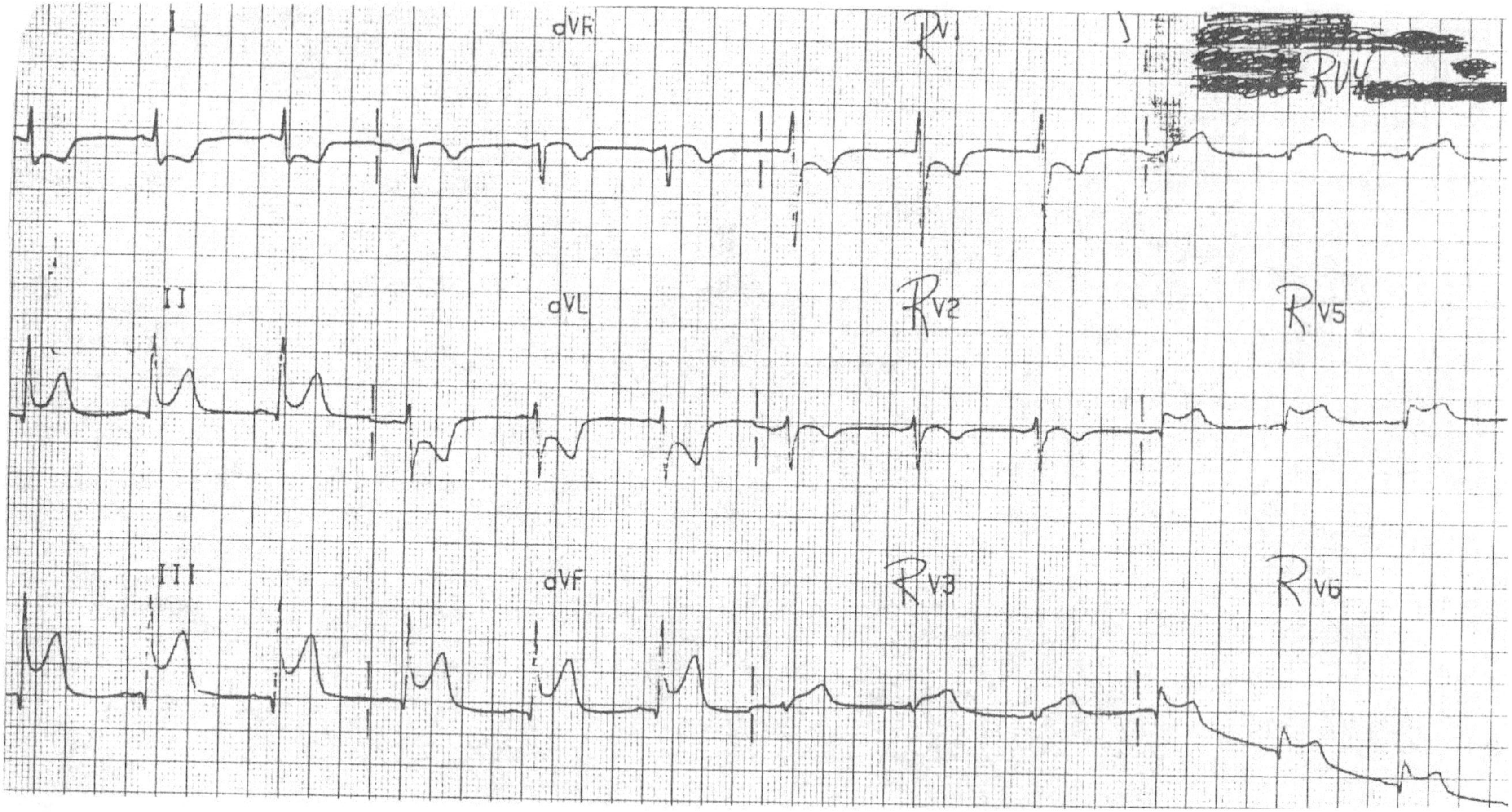

Exercise #8

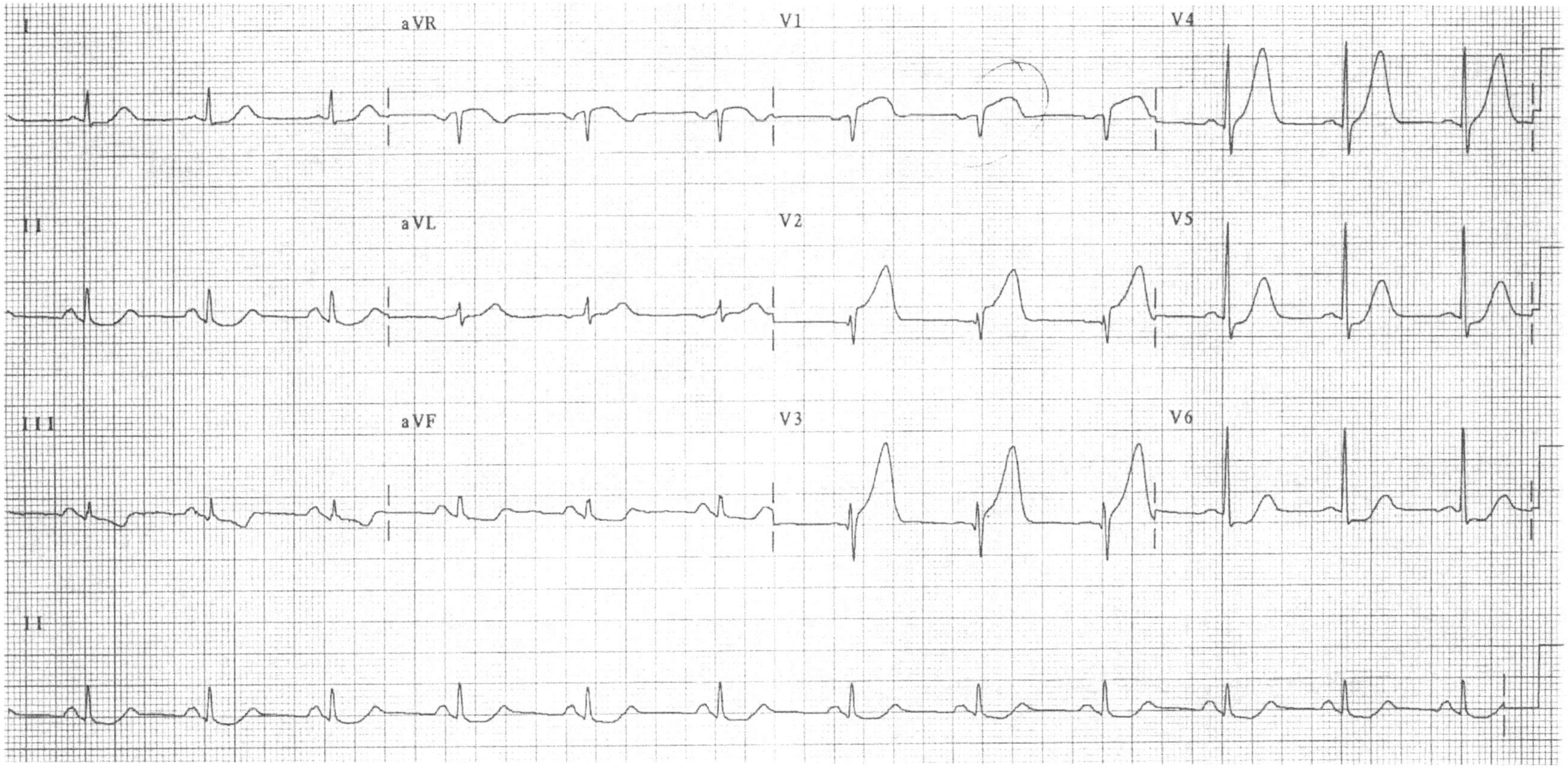

p.46

Exercise #9

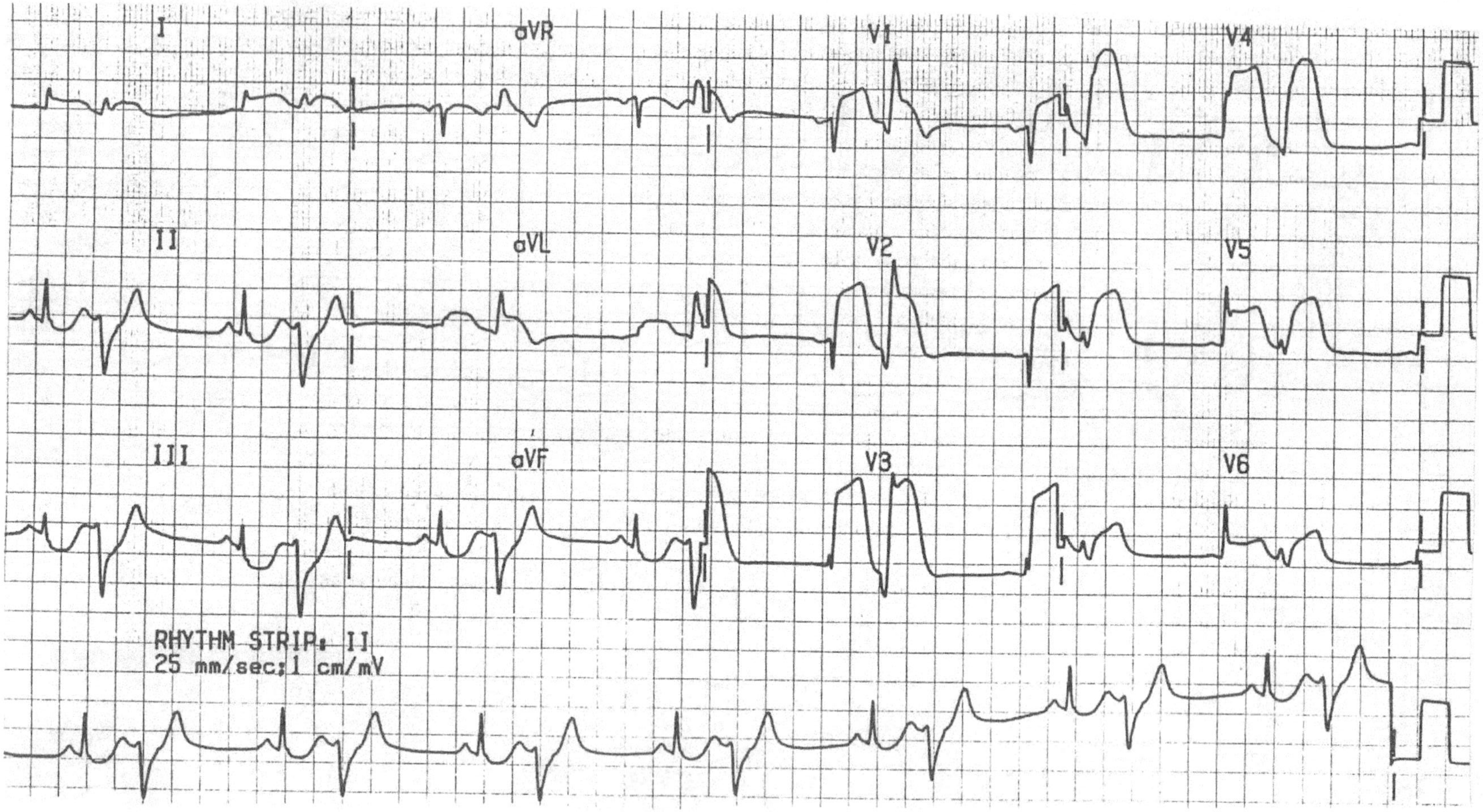

Exercise #10

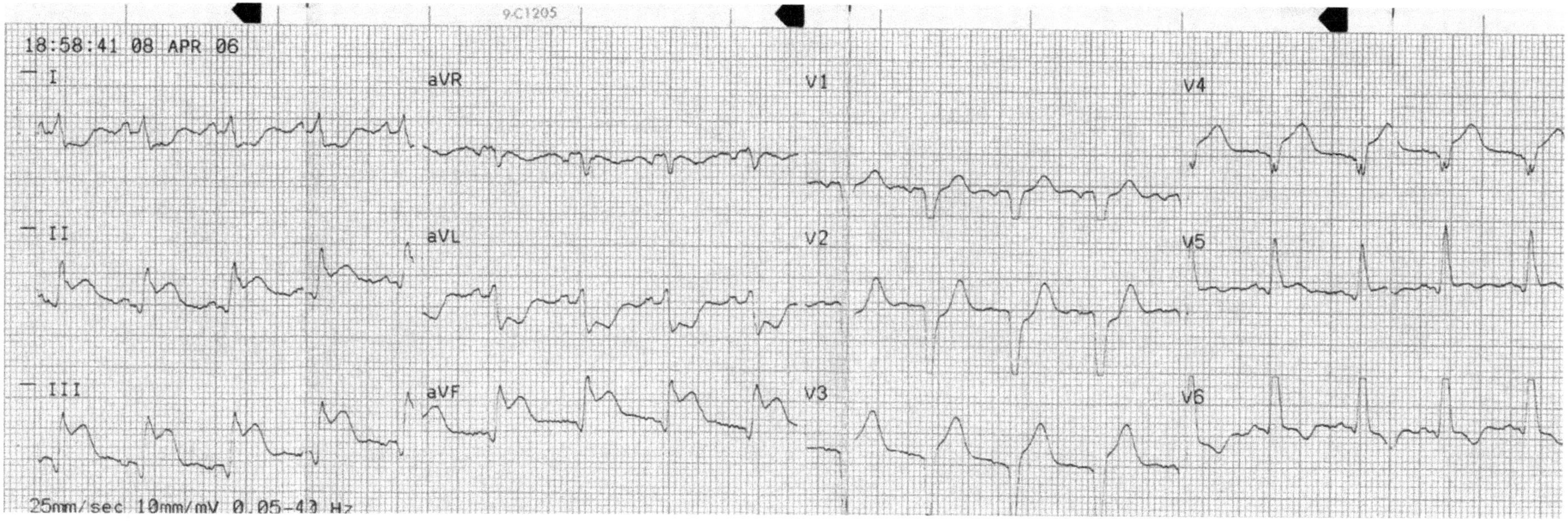

p.48

The Great Impostors

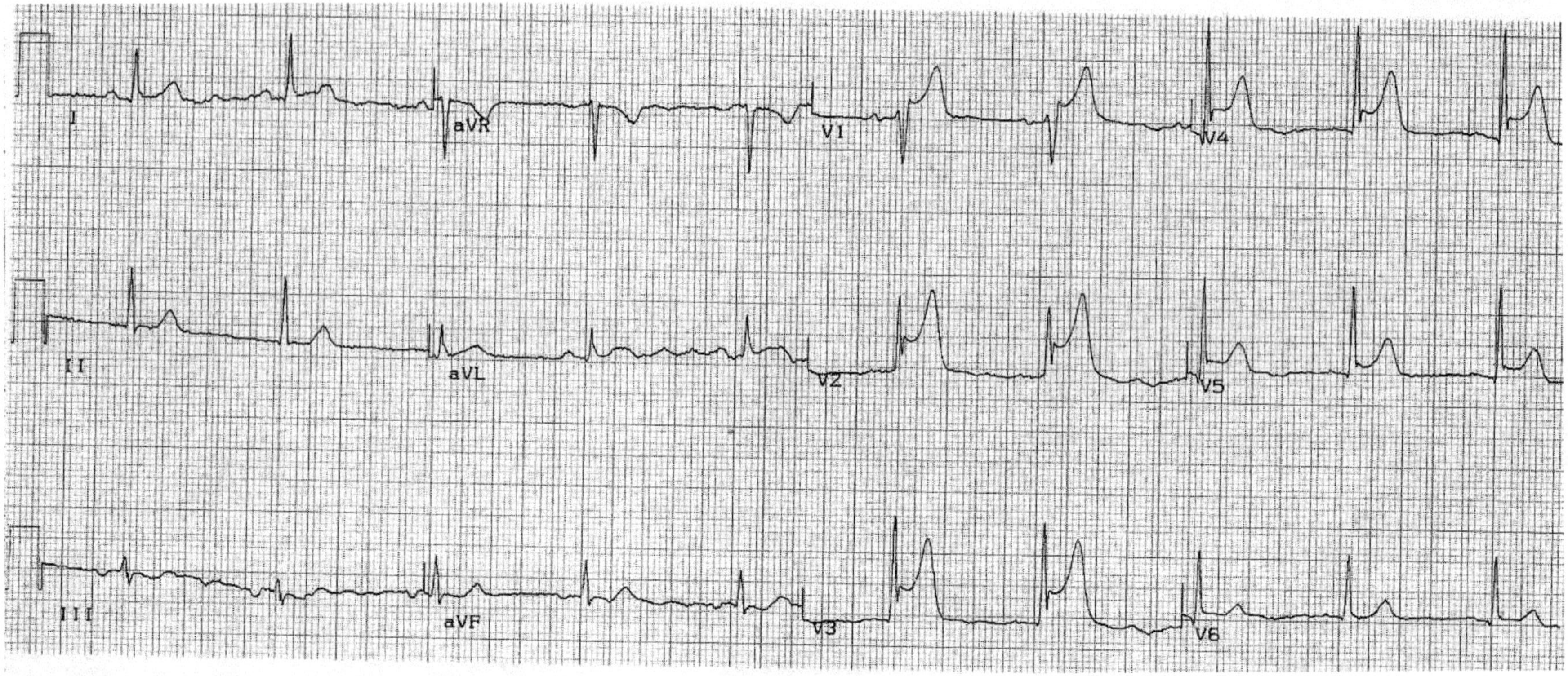

p.49

The Great Impostors

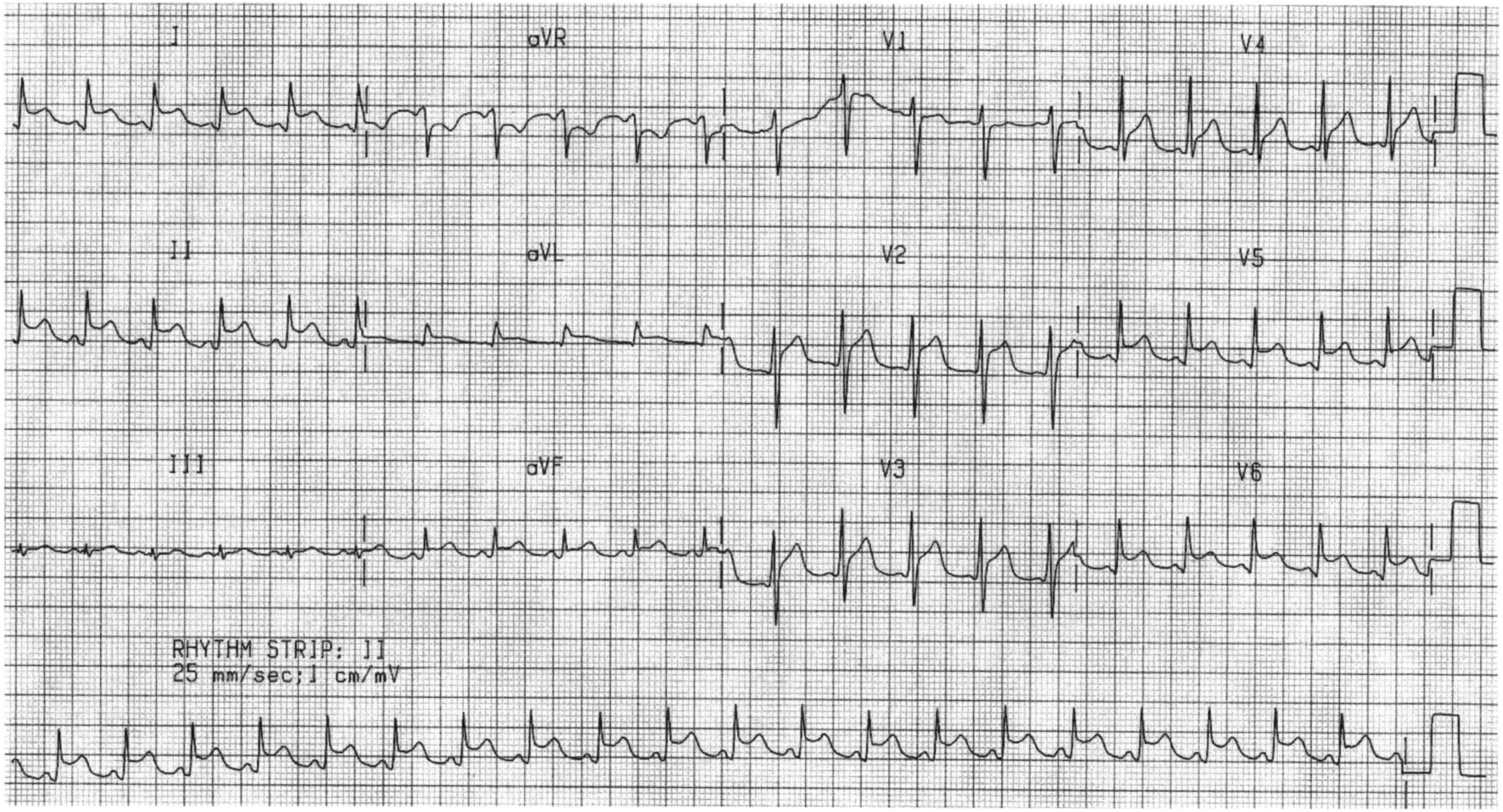

The Great Impostors

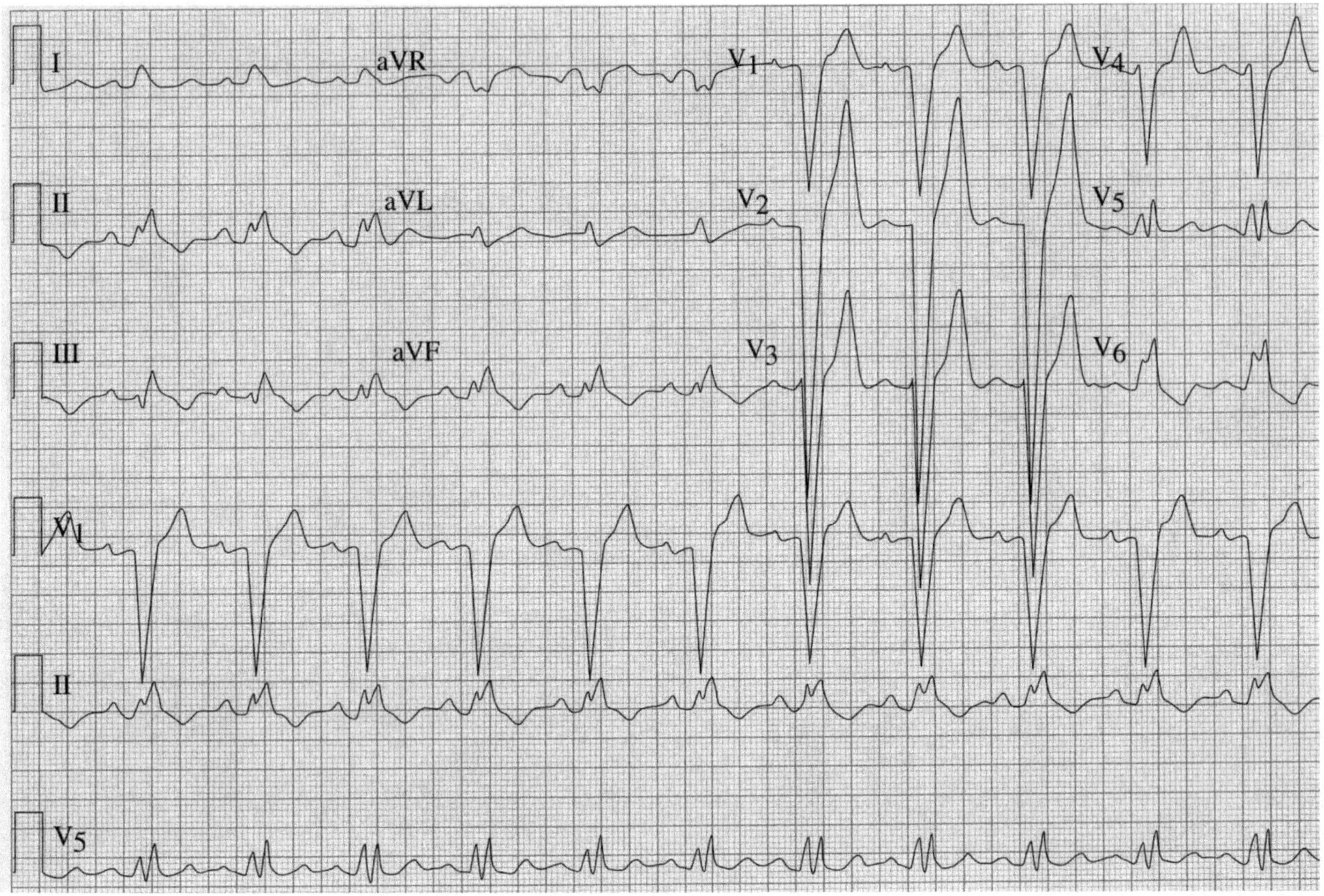

p.51

APPENDIX

Vector/Axis estimation

What is axis?

Current flows through the heart in many directions. If conduction is normal, an impulse will begin at the SA node, spread across both atria, pause at the AV node briefly, then spread across both ventricles simultaneously.

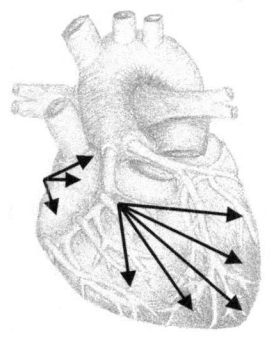

- Since the left ventricle of thicker than the right ventricle, there is logically more electrical activity on the left side of the heart compared with the right side.

- Axis is the summary of all waves of depolarization - also referred to as "vector".

Why Estimate Axis?

General rules

- For your brain only (FYBO)
- Axis moves away from infarction (generally)
- Axis moves toward hypertrophy

Specific Rules - Left Axis Deviation

- pregnancy, obesity or ascites
- left ventricular hypertrophy
- anterior MI (questionable value?)
- inferior MI
- aberrant ventricular conduction
- left anterior hemiblock

Specific Rules - Right Axis Deviation

- normal finding in children
- left posterior hemiblock
- anterior MI (questionable value?)
- lateral MI
- *aberrant ventricular conduction*
- right ventricular hypertrophy

Specific Rules - No Man's Land (extreme right axis deviation)

- *ventricular tachycardia*
- aneurysm of the left ventricle
- ectopic ventricular impulse
- ventricular pacing

Steps to Determine Axis
EASIER ALTERNATIVE - LESS ACCURATE

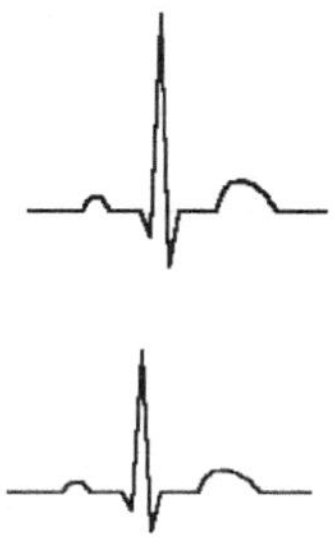

	If Lead I is +ve and Lead aVF is also +ve	Normal Axis
	If Lead I is +ve and Lead aVF is –ve *And Lead II is -ve*	Left Axis Deviation
	If Lead I is -ve and Lead aVF is +ve *And Lead II is -ve*	Right Axis Deviation
	If Lead I is -ve and Lead aVF is also -ve	Extreme Right Axis Deviation "No Man's Land"

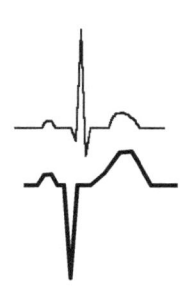

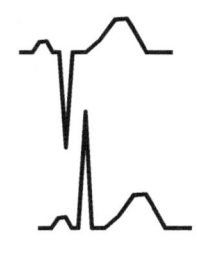

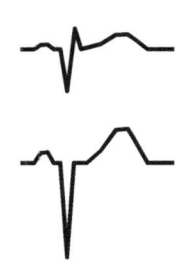

p.54

Notes

REFERENCES

1. (2008). Statistics - Heart and Stroke Foundation of Canada. Retrieved from http://www.heartandstroke.com/site/c.ikIQLcMWJtE/b.3483991/

2. (2006). CDC - DHDSP - Heart Disease Facts. Retrieved from http://www.cdc.gov/heartdisease/facts.htm

3. Fenton, D.E., (2005): **Myocardial Infarction**. eMedicine. Retrieved from: http://www.emedicine.com/EMERG/topic327.htm

4. Maloba, M (2004): **Pre-Hospital ECG. Effect on door to needle time and overall pain to needle time.** Best Evidence Topics. http://www.bestbets.org/cgi-bin/bets.pl?record=00765

5. Morrison LJ, Brooks S, Sawadsky B, McDonald A, Verbeek PR. (2006, Dec.): **Prehospital 12-lead electrocardiography impact on acute myocardial infarction treatment times and mortality: a systematic review.** Academic Emergency Medicine. 2006 Jan;13(1):84-9.

6. Aufderheide, T.P., Benner, J.P., Brady, W.J., Braithwaite, S., Currance, S.B., Ferguson, J.D., Kielar, N.D., Perron, A.D., (2003 Mar): **The prehospital 12-lead electrocardiogram: impact on management of the out-of-hospital acute coronary syndrome patient.** American Journal of Emergency Medicine. 21(2):136-42

7. Anderson PD, Mitchell PM, Rathlev NK, Fish SS, Feldman JA. (Nov., 2004): **Potential diversion rates associated with prehospital acute myocardial infarction triage strategies**. The Journal of Emergency Medicine. 27(4):345-53

8. Smalling RW, Giesler G. (2003, Spring): **The level I cardiovascular center: is it time?** The American Heart Hospital Journal. 1(2):170-4

9. Hunt. A., Jacobs, A.K. (2004): **ACC/AHA Guidelines for the Management of Patients With ST-Elevation Myocardial.** 110;82-292

10. Frascone, R.J., Provo, T.A.: **12-lead Electrocardiograms During Basic Life Support Care**. Prehospital Emergency Care. 2004 Apr-Jun;8(2):212-6.

11. Tomoyuki Hori, Toshiro Kurosawa, Makoto Yoshida, Masaru Yamazoe, Yoshifusa Aizawa, Tohru Izumi: **Factors Predicting Mortality in Patients after Myocardial Infarction Caused by Left Main Coronary Artery Occlusion: Significance of ST Segment Elevation in Both aVR and aVL Leads** Japanese Heart Journal. Vol. 41 (2000) , No. 5 pp.571-581

RECOMMENDED READING/WEBSITES

Dr Smith's ECG blog
http://hqmeded-ecg.blogspot.ca/

Dr Amal Mattu's Emergency ECG Video of the Week
http://ekgumem.tumblr.com/

Tom Bouthillet's EMS 12 Lead
http://www.ems12lead.com/

Dr. Ken Graur ECG Interpretation
http://ecg-interpretation.blogspot.ca/

If you're looking for more detail on 12 Lead ECG interpretation, I recommend Dr. Grauer's books. They are superb!

Michelle Cleland RN, MSN(c), CCN(C), CNCC(C), CNN(C)
Acute Care Education: www.ace.cc

About the author

Rob Theriault BHSc., EMCA, RCT(Adv.), CCP(F)

Rob Theriault has been in the Emergency Medical Services (EMS) industry since 1984, and while he continues to work part-time as an Advanced Care Paramedic in the field, he is a full time professor of paramedicine at Georgian College in Ontario, Canada. Rob trained as a Cardiology Technologist and started teaching ECG interpretation in the 1980s. He received his Bachelor of Health Sciences Degree in Paramedicine from Victoria University in Melbourne, Australia. Rob is also the Past President of the Ontario Paramedic Association and is the Lead on the provincial application for paramedic self-regulation.

From 1987-1997, Rob worked on the Ontario Ministry of Health Air Ambulance helicopter "Bandage One", now known as "Ornge". There, Rob trained as a Critical Care Flight Paramedic. With over a decade as a flight paramedic, Rob looked after some of the most critically ill and injured patients in the province. In recognition of Rob's expertise, he was assigned as personal paramedic to two former U.S. Presidents and in 1995 was featured in the award winning Discovery Channel series "FlightPath: Bandage One".

Rob is both a published and self-published author, researcher, blogger, Podcaster and speaks at conferences across Canada and around the world. He is also a recipient of the Ontario Colleges "Innovative Teaching with Technology Award" for his use of technology to enhance learning, the Governor General of Canada EMS Exemplary Service medal and the Queen Elizabeth II Diamond Jubilee medal for his influence on the Canadian EMS system as a paramedic educator, author and public speaker.

CPSIA information can be obtained
at www.ICGtesting.com
Printed in the USA
LVHW062239090123
736733LV00004B/425

9 780993 686023